Legal and Ethical Issues in Physical Therapy

Legal and Ethical Issues in Physical Therapy

Laura Lee Swisher, M.Div., P.T.

Clinical Coordinator, Subacute Unit, Department of Rehabilitation Services, Vanderbilt University Medical Center, Nashville, Tennessee

Carol Krueger-Brophy, J.D., P.T.

Staff Physical Therapist, Baptist Hospital, Nashville, Tennessee; Adjunct Assistant Professor, Tennessee State University, Nashville

Butterworth–Heinemann

Boston   Oxford   Johannesburg   Melbourne   New Delhi   Singapore

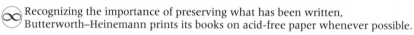

Butterworth–Heinemann supports the efforts of American Forests and the Global ReLeaf program in its campaign for the betterment of trees, forests, and our environment.

Library of Congress Cataloging-in-Publication Data

Swisher, Laura L.
    Legal and ethical issues in physical therapy / Laura L. Swisher,
Carol Krueger-Brophy.
        p.   cm.
    Includes bibliographical references and index.
    ISBN 0-7506-9788-1
    1. Physical therapists--Legal status, laws, etc.--United States.
    2. Medical ethics--United States.   I. Krueger-Brophy, Carol.
    II. Title.
    KF2915.T 452S93   1997
    174'.2--dc21   97-23859
                                                                CIP

British Library Cataloguing-in-Publication Data
A catalogue record for this book is available from the British Library.

The publisher offers special discounts on bulk orders of this book.

For information, please contact:
Manager of Special Sales
Butterworth–Heinemann
225 Wildwood Avenue
Woburn, MA 01801-2041
Tel: 781-904-2500
Fax: 781-904-2620

For information on all Butterworth–Heinemann publications available,
contact our World Wide Web home page at: http://www.bh.com

10 9 8 7 6 5 4 3 2 1

Printed in the United States of America

For Dean, Mary Lee, and Marsha, who taught me many lessons about ethics, wisdom, virtue, and integrity

L.L.S.

To Sean, with love, respect, admiration, and gratitude

C.K.B.

Contents

Preface

This book provides an introduction to legal and ethical issues faced by physical therapists in a variety of practice settings. These issues demonstrate the complexity and richness of the ethical and legal problems encountered. We do not intend to address each potential issue that may arise in a clinical setting. Rather, the issues presented introduce readers to ways of thinking about and tools for devising solutions to problems in law and ethics.

Chapter 1 lays the groundwork for legal and ethical problem solving. We describe legal and regulatory influences on physical therapy practice. We discuss various principles and approaches used in ethical decision making, and propose a framework for ethical analysis. In addition, Chapter 1 clarifies the similarities and distinctions between law, ethics, and medicine and describes certain unique aspects of the health care environment that affect legal and ethical analysis.

Each chapter presents cases involving legal and ethical considerations. We elaborate on issues posed by the cases and apply legal and ethical principles to the problems. The chapters conclude with notes and questions to assist readers in making cross references and developing basic skills in ethical and legal issue spotting and problem solving. No right or wrong answers are provided; a single correct course of action is rarely apparent, and numerous factors, including variations in state law, may alter outcomes at different facilities. Ethical and legal problems are posed in a variety of practice settings; this is not to suggest that particular issues will arise only within a certain setting. We believe that this case-oriented framework enhances learning and facilitates recognition of legal and ethical problems and solutions in the practice setting.

Chapter 7 discusses where and when to turn for assistance in formulating possible solutions to ethical and legal problems and describes phases and types of litigation that a therapist might encounter. Readers are cautioned that this work does not offer legal advice per se; therapists faced with legal questions must consult facility or private attorneys. This work illustrates when such consultation may be advisable.

The intended audience includes physical therapists in clinical practice or administration as well as physical therapy students beginning clinical experience. Physical therapists are increasingly functioning as independent professionals within the health care community and need to be aware of the responsibilities and liabilities associated with professional autonomy.

This work is the first of its kind, as it integrates law and ethics specifically within the physical therapy context. We believe that such treatment of these topics is essential, as focus on a single aspect of a multilayered problem may create serious repercussions for patients and practitioners.

L.L.S.
C.K.B.

Acknowledgments

With special appreciation to the colleagues who reviewed this work: Dr. James Hays, Pat Fleming, Ann Giffin, and Maryellen Maley.

Legal and Ethical Issues in Physical Therapy

1

Introduction to Legal
and Ethical Principles

This introduction provides the background necessary for consideration of legal and ethical problems. This chapter discusses legal and regulatory influences on the practice of physical therapy; the field of medical ethics and a framework for ethical decision making; several similarities and distinctions among law, ethics, and medicine; and several unique features of the clinical environment and of the broader health care environment that add complexity to legal and ethical analysis.

LEGAL AND REGULATORY INFLUENCES

Health care professionals, including physical therapists (PTs), are subject to a web of legal and regulatory influences, both public and private. Ethical issues are frequently interwoven with legal issues. Figure 1.1 presents a graphic representation of some of the legal and regulatory influences encountered in physical therapy practice.

Sources of Law

The first authority that health care professionals are subject to is laws. Laws may be legislatively created at both the federal and state levels and are called *statutes*. An example of a law created at the federal level is the Health Care Quality Improvement Act (HCQIA), which addresses peer review standards and mandates creation of the National Practitioner Data Bank.[1] At the state level, many jurisdictions have specific statutes regarding medical malpractice suits and tort reform efforts. Physical therapy practice acts are also a creation of state law.

In addition to laws created by statute, some legal principles, known as *case law* or *common law*, are set forth in decisions by both state and federal judges. Federal cases interpreting the HCQIA are beginning to

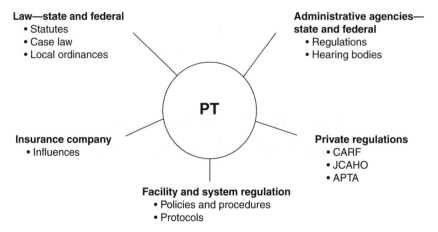

Figure 1.1 Legal and regulatory influences encountered in physical therapy practice. (PT = physical therapist; CARF = Commission on Accreditation of Rehabilitation Facilities; JCAHO = Joint Commission on Accreditation of Healthcare Organizations; APTA = American Physical Therapy Association.)

appear. For example, hospitals have been granted immunity as a matter of law in medical staff privilege termination cases if they can show that they have met the requirements of the HCQIA in their peer review proceedings.[2] State cases that address contributory or comparative negligence—that is, determining whether a malpractice plaintiff can recover damages if the plaintiff was partially at fault for the injury—are examples of state case law.

A state's attorney general may be asked to issue an advisory opinion regarding the meaning of a particular law that has been called into question or that is subject to several interpretations. In Tennessee, the attorney general provided an interpretation of a physician ban on self-referrals, suggesting that the law would apply to payment of a percentage of gross collections to an independent practice management company.[3]

The question of whether an issue is governed by state or federal law is often complex, subject itself to litigation, and beyond the scope of this work. In brief, certain matters, such as constitutional law questions, are generally considered federal matters (although state constitutions often also address issues involving fundamental rights). Federal courts also consider cases involving federal statutes or disputes between citizens of different states (if the amount in question exceeds a certain threshold). Historically, other matters, such as licensure of health care professionals, have been left to the states, subject to certain constitutional limitations.[4]

Finally, local communities may have ordinances enacted by the city council or other governing body that affect PTs. An example is a local building code that specifies requirements for the electrical system in a physical therapy clinic. If a clinic were found to be in violation of the code and an injury resulted, a plaintiff might present evidence of the code violation to show that the therapist was negligent in not meeting the city requirements.

Administrative Law

Administrative agencies, both state and federal, are critical in determining how a particular statute is interpreted by issuing regulations and by acting as quasi-judicial hearing bodies; this is known as *administrative law*. Typically, authority is expressly delegated to the agencies by statute to act on behalf of the legislature in these areas. Regulations provide additional specific guidance in interpreting statutes. Once adopted, such regulations generally have the force of law and are enforced as if adopted by the legislature. For example, the Health Care Financing Administration issued regulations in 1995 interpreting portions of the Omnibus Budget Reconciliation Acts (OBRA) of 1989, 1990, and 1993 and the Social Security Act Amendments of 1994, which deal with the financial relationship between physicians and referrals to providers of clinical laboratory services.[5] State agencies also often issue regulations that set forth specifics regarding practice issues, or they delegate their power to do so to specially created boards. In Tennessee, for example, the state board of physical and occupational therapy examiners has issued rules and regulations defining direct supervision by PTs.[6]

Federal agencies that affect the provision of health care in the United States include the Department of Health and Human Services (HHS) and its subsidiary, the Health Care Financing Agency; the Food and Drug Administration; the Social Security Administration; and the Federal Trade Commission (note that this is not an exhaustive list). HHS regulates and oversees federal health care programs such as Medicare and Medicaid. The Health Care Financing Agency controls regulatory aspects of funding for these programs. The Food and Drug Administration is charged with overseeing entry of new medical devices and pharmaceuticals into the health care market. The Social Security Administration makes determinations about an individual's eligibility for certain disability benefits. The role of the Federal Trade Commission is to promote free competition and to provide protection against unfair trade practices.

In addition to issuing regulations, federal and state agencies may act as hearing bodies, considering cases that fall within their regulatory purview. For example, federal administrative law judges consider appeals from people who have been determined ineligible for social security disability benefits. State licensure boards act as hearing bodies in cases involving infringements of the state practice act. There is usually a right to judicial review of these administrative proceedings after administrative remedies have been exhausted.

Private Regulation

In addition to these legal and regulatory authorities, private regulators play an increasingly important role in ensuring physical therapy compliance with practice standards. Private agencies include the Commission on Accreditation of Rehabilitation Facilities (CARF), the Joint Commission on Accreditation of Healthcare Organizations (JCAHO), and the American Physical Therapy Association (APTA). Both CARF and JCAHO focus primarily on facility standards, although certain portions of the standards, such as those dealing with documentation, have implications for individual professional practice.

The APTA, through its *Guide for Professional Conduct* and the *Standards of Practice,* sets forth explicit ethical rules that its members must comply with to retain membership. In addition, practice parameters developed through APTA initiatives may help to define specific clinical aspects of care.[7]

Facility and System Regulation

Health care facilities and integrated health care systems also establish particular rules for their professional employees and member facilities. These rules might include medical staff bylaws, facility and department policies and procedures, or critical pathways.

Insurance Company Influences

Although third-party payers are not regulators per se, their requirements are now de facto types of regulations that must be met to ensure reimbursement. Some insurers require a specific frequency or form of documentation. Managed care contracts sometimes impose explicit guidelines on providers, demanding adherence to particular procedures and standards. In addition to requiring information and compliance with standards, insurance companies have assumed an investigative role in such matters as health care fraud and abuse. Claims information and supporting documentation are scrutinized for outliers and patterns suggesting an intent to defraud the insurance company. The growth of this type of oversight has skyrocketed in recent years as companies seek to control medical costs.

Interplay Between Legal and Regulatory Authorities

Each of these legal and regulatory influences operates concurrently to control health care practice. A state or federal legislature may enact a statute that is then interpreted by the corresponding agency; then the statute or regulations may be interpreted by a judge through case law; such case interpretations might then be overturned through new legislation. The process is dynamic rather than static.

It is important to note that each of the legal and regulatory authorities described is able to impose separate sanctions arising from the same course of conduct. An individual found guilty of violating the federal antikickback statute, for example, may receive a federal sentence and fine, be excluded from participation as a provider of services under Medicare and Medicaid, lose state licensure, be suspended by the APTA, lose a hospital position, and face cancellation of managed care contracts.

INTRODUCTION TO ETHICAL CONCEPTS

Whereas legal standards and laws are set by legislative authorities and interpreted by judicial bodies, moral and ethical standards are developed within communities or organizations and enforced through education and persuasion. The interpreters and analysts of ethical standards have traditionally been philosophers and theologians. This section describes the origin and components of ethics, the major schools of ethics, and the development of ethics in medicine.

What Is Ethics?

Ethics developed as a field of *philosophy* that deals with moral conduct. In fact, ethics is sometimes referred to as *moral philosophy*.[8] Ethics involves philosophical reflection on questions of right or wrong. Jacques Thiroux's[9] definition is helpful in this regard:

> Ethics ... deals with what is right or wrong in human behavior and conduct. It asks such questions as what constitutes any person or action being good, bad, right, or wrong, and how do we know (epistemology)? What part does self-interest or the interests of others play in making moral decisions and judgments? What theories of conduct are valid or invalid and why? Should we use principles or rules or laws, or should we let each situation decide our morality? Are killing, lying, cheating, stealing, and sexual acts right or wrong, and why or why not?

Although the terms *ethics, ethical, moral,* and *morality,* and the terms *immoral,* and *unethical* are used interchangeably[9] in common parlance, many philosophers make a distinction between ethics and morality. "To them *morality* refers to human conduct and values, and *ethics* refers to the study of those areas."[10] A distinction between ethics and morality suggests that morality is the entire constellation of laws, values, and guidelines that are promulgated by a culture or society and may become internalized by an individual.[8] These sanctions place different levels of demands on individuals. According to Frankena[8]:

> Considered as a social system of regulation, morality is like law on the one hand and convention or etiquette on the other.... But convention does not deal with matters of such crucial social importance as those dealt with by law and morality; it seems to rest largely on considerations of appearance, taste, and convenience.

These levels of morality undergird the wide range of the use of the words *wrong, unethical,* or *immoral.* Although someone might say that it is wrong to wear denim jeans to a formal reception at the White House, this violation of conventional etiquette is not on the same level of immorality as theft or murder.

In contrast to this nearly unconscious or preconscious realm of morality, ethics involves "systematic reflection on and [rational] analysis of morality."[11] The study of ethics can be divided into three types of approaches: scientific or descriptive, normative or prescriptive, and metaethical or analytic.* In scientific ethics, empirical methods are used to study the moral behavior or customs of a particular society or group of people.[8, 9] Normative ethics is concerned with what individuals should or ought to do. Metaethics goes beyond (*meta* is Greek for beyond) normative ethics and attempts to form a rational justification for moral judgments. On which criteria should ethical judgments be based? Metaethics is also concerned with the meaning and use of ethical terms such as *good* and *ethical.*[8] In practice it is impossible to consider normative ethics without considering both descriptive and metaethical ethics. Individuals cannot make decisions about what they ought to do without understanding the moral context of a specific cultural tradition and without raising questions about the meaning of ethical terms in general.

The main concern of this book is to examine legal and ethical issues involved in the practice of physical therapy. This book, therefore, is concerned mainly with normative or prescriptive ethics of the profession of physical therapy, or *applied ethics.* Examination of these issues

---

*There are a number of approaches to categorizing ethics. Purtilo describes two (normative and metaethical); Frankena uses three; Thiroux uses two: descriptive/scientific and philosophical, which he subdivides into two subcategories (normative and metaethical).

may raise both descriptive and metaethical issues, but the main concern is for prescriptive ethics.

Traditional Ethical Concepts

Ethics traditionally has dealt with certain categories, "elements,"* or norms used in ethical reflection. These categories are

1. Duties, rights, and obligations
2. Consequences
3. Virtue or character
4. Context, environment, and situation
5. Values†

Each of these categories has been emphasized by a particular normative theory as the basis for all ethical decisions.

Duties, Rights, and Obligations

Duties are moral responsibilities or demands.[10] Some of these duties or obligations stem from specific social relationships. Parents have certain obligations and duties to their children, such as protection from harm and provision of food and clothing. PTs have specific obligations that stem from the relationships and duties involved in their work. Maintaining confidentiality is an example of this kind of duty. Other duties do not arise from specific relationships but rather reflect timeless and universal obligations for other human beings. Justice and the prohibitions of the Ten Commandments are examples of this kind of duty. Duties of this nature are described as *deontological* (from *ontos,* the Greek root for duty) because they seem to come from a higher being or merely by virtue of human existence. These obligations are not contingent on particular circumstances or relationships but are always "right."

Some philosophers have argued that all ethical decisions are determined by duties and rules that describe those obligations. The most well-known representative of this school is Immanuel Kant (1724–1804),[12] who argued that universal principles of morality can be derived a priori from reason. Kant believed that people should act in such a way that moral actions can be universalized, a principle that he called the *categorical imperative*—that is, people should act in such a way that an action could become a universal law.[10] Expressed differently,

---

*Purtilo uses this chemical term to refer to principles or norms in ethics.

†Values cut across all categories. Although value is not usually considered a separate category of analysis, it is helpful to focus on this category on its own.

the categorical imperative states that everyone should always treat fellow human beings as ends in themselves rather than as means only.

Kant's emphasis on duties and obligations as the primary considerations leaves little room for the consideration of consequences in determining right or wrong action. Deontological frameworks, such as Kant's, also have difficulty dealing with situations in which duties seem to conflict, as Kant's own example illustrates: Suppose that a murderer were to come to your door looking for your friend, who is upstairs in your home.[10, 12] The murderer asks if you know where your friend is. Is it right to lie to the murderer? The case presents a conflict between the obligation to tell the truth and the obligation to prevent harm to the friend. (However, note that the dilemma within this situation revolves around the presumed consequence of harm being done to your friend.) Kant reasoned that it would be wrong to lie because truth is a universal obligation and the conduct of lying cannot be universalized. The example indirectly poses the question as to what kind of world would result if individuals failed to tell the truth whenever they projected a negative consequence to their actions.

W.D. Ross (1877–1971) attempted to address the problem of conflicting obligations by distinguishing prima facie obligations from actual or absolute obligations.[13] "A prima facie obligation is simply an obligation that can be overridden by a more important obligation."[10] When one obligation conflicts with another obligation, an individual must make a moral judgment as to which obligation is prima facie and which must be honored in a given situation. In other words, a prima facie obligation is not binding only because there is a more important, pressing obligation in that situation. If Kant's dilemma is considered from the standpoint of Ross's prima facie and actual duties, Ross would argue that telling the truth in this situation is a prima facie obligation that would be subordinate to the obligation to prevent harm to the friend.[10]

A corollary of the concept of duty is the concept of rights. "Broadly defined, a *right* is an entitlement to act or have others act in a certain way. The connection between rights and duties is that, generally speaking, if you have a right to do something, then someone else has a correlative duty to act in a certain way."[10] For example, if a patient has the right to be informed of the risks associated with treatment, then the health care provider has the duty to disclose those risks. The correlative relationship between rights and duties has important implications for the idea of health care as a right.

Consequences

Another element considered in moral judgments is the effect or consequences that an individual's actions have on others. One major school of thinking, consequentialism, emphasizes consequences rather than duties in determining which actions are morally correct. This approach to ethics is also called *teleological* (from the Greek word for end), because it emphasizes the outcomes or results of actions. Utilitarianism is the most well-known example of consequentialist ethical theory. Developed by Jeremy Bentham (1748–1832) and John Stuart Mill (1806–1873), utilitarianism is commonly characterized as advocating the greatest good for the greatest number. Frankena[8] described utilitarianism in this manner:

> There are less precise ways of defining utilitarianism, which I shall use for convenience, but in my own use of the term, I shall mean the view that the sole ultimate standard of right, wrong, and obligation is the *principle of utility*, which says quite strictly that the moral end to be sought in all we do is *the greatest possible balance of good over evil* (or the least possible balance of evil over good) in the world as a whole. Here "good" and "evil" mean nonmoral good and evil. This implies that whatever the good and the bad are, they are capable of being measured and balanced against each other in some quantitative or at least mathematical way.

Act utilitarians believe that the greatest good should be calculated for every action (frequently through cost-benefit analysis). *Rule utilitarians*, on the other hand, believe that individuals should follow rules that promote the greatest good. For example, rule utilitarians might support a rule that prohibits killing except in self-defense.[9] One obvious drawback to utilitarianism is the difficulty of calculating the effects of actions. Although a good deal of time can be spent projecting consequences of actions, there is no real way of determining the long-term consequences of much of what an individual does. In contrast to the Kantian deontological consideration of the moral worth of each individual, utilitarianism has difficulty protecting individual worth and rights.

Virtue

In addition to the principles and rules for behavior emphasized by traditional ethics, another important consideration in an ethical decision is the character or virtue of the individual performing the act. Alasdair MacIntyre[14] defined three different approaches to virtue:

> We thus have at least three very different conceptions of a virtue to confront: a virtue is a quality which enables an individual to discharge his or her social role (Homer); a virtue is a quality which enables an individual to move towards the achievement of the specifically human *telos*, whether natural or supernatural (Aristotle, the New Testament and Aquinas); a virtue is a quality which has utility in achieving earthly and heavenly success (Franklin).

Aristotle's (384–322 BC) ethical system was organized entirely around the practice of virtues. Aristotelian ethics focused on becoming a morally good person through the development of personal characteristics or traits that he called virtues. According to Aristotle, human beings have a natural capacity for ethical behavior,[9] and the development of that ethical nature demands practice. Through practice, the habit of morality is acquired, which is the proper exercise of virtue.

Virtue, or character, ethics provides an important complement to duty-based and consequentialist normative theories. While duty, or consequentialist,* ethics asks "What shall we do?" virtue-based theories pose the question "What kind of person shall I be?" In reality, individuals cannot expect to perform moral acts unless they have acquired moral character developed by the practice of the virtues.

Because of its interest in the process and goal of developing moral persons, virtue-based ethics also indirectly emphasizes the role of community and social systems. For this reason, the virtue-based perspective is congruent with communitarian approaches, which emphasize the community or social goals.

Alasdair MacIntyre's work represents an excellent example of a communitarian approach built on virtue. In *After Virtue*, MacIntyre described the limitations of democratic liberalism, which emphasizes individual rights. In American society, which is dominated by rights, "[t]here seems to be no rational way of securing moral agreement in our culture," according to MacIntyre.[14] He saw this illustrated by the nature of contemporary moral debates, which he described as interminable, in which the participants advance viewpoints based on incompatible or incommensurable notions of particular values. As MacIntyre noted, there seems to be no way to resolve these sorts of conflicts in American society.[14]

This development, in MacIntyre's opinion, represents the inability of liberal individualism to sustain a viable notion of community. "For liberal individualism a community is simply an arena in which individuals each pursue their own self-chosen conception of the good life, and political institutions exist to provide that degree of order which makes such self-determined activity possible."[14] In part, this is a result of the emphasis on universal principles of ethical analysis without any relationship to the moral life of the community.

For MacIntyre, the alternative to liberal individualism is a return to Aristotle's virtue-based communitarian ethics. From the Aristotelian standpoint, every species has its own nature and, therefore, its own telos, or purpose. Doing the good is therefore moving toward that

---

*Aristotle's ethical system has also been regarded as a teleological system because it is oriented toward an end: the development of a moral person and what Aristotle called happiness. However, this telos, or purpose, differs from focusing on consequences of actions.

innate purpose. The good for human beings is what Aristotle called *eudaimonia* (happiness or prosperity).[14] "The virtues are precisely those qualities the possession of which will enable an individual to achieve *eudaimonia* and the lack of which will frustrate his movement toward that *telos*."[14] From Aristotle's perspective, human beings are essentially political. Accordingly, each individual's good is inherently related to the good of the community. The idea of conflict between self-interest and the common good is inconceivable from an Aristotelian perspective. Virtues are the means by which individuals achieve both happiness and the common good.

Aristotle's virtue-based ethics is very different from current ethical thought in that it places very little emphasis on rules for behavior.[14] As MacIntyre noted, this diverges sharply from the liberal democratic-bureaucratic tradition, which emphasizes rules of conduct. Without a concept of the common good, the liberal democratic tradition has demonstrated an inability to resolve ethical debates. If one argues for justice out of self-interest and another argues for liberty out of self-interest, then arguments may be essentially incommensurable.[14]

The health care reform debates of the early 1990s are examples of incommensurable arguments. Surveys of public opinion demonstrate that many Americans oppose Medicare cuts but also support reducing the deficit. There seems to be no way for American society to tie together beliefs about individuals' rights and access to health care and the common good. MacIntyre's critique suggests a re-emphasis on virtues within the context of the common good. It does not suggest a vehicle for bridging the gap between a pluralistic society of competing interests and a unitary society working toward a common good.

Context, Environment, and Situation

Kant argued that moral principles ought to be capable of universal application. Principles are by their very nature general. There should be no surprise that application of general ethical principles to specific circumstances is difficult; often yielding conflict between the principles. How do individuals decide which principle is most important when principles or rules conflict? One important factor, although not the only factor, in determining that decision is the context or environment.

Context addresses what is appropriate or fitting in a particular culture, setting, or situation. For example, in our culture, it is not considered appropriate to eat with one's fingers at a formal dinner. Good moral decisions, actions, and traits take into account the specific moral and historical contexts in which they occur. For example, the distinction between the character traits (virtues) of arrogance and self-assurance must in part be determined by the context in which they occur. Similarly, context influences the interpretation of actions that violate rules of conduct. If my car strikes a pedestrian after a truck slams into the rear of my car, I would not likely be charged with murder. However, if I had consumed a six-pack of beer before driving erratically, I could be guilty of murder.

In *Ethics and the Clinical Encounter,* Richard Zaner[15] argued that the failure of biomedical ethics resides in part in its inability to understand the clinical context or the clinical relationships that characterize medical settings. By restricting discussions to the traditional principles (autonomy, beneficence, nonmaleficence, and justice), attention is diverted from the specific context of the medical facts on which the case turns.

> It ought to be clear that restricting moral discourse to the formal level of principles, or that of social policy, fails in several ways to be responsive to the real, clinical demands of such a case.... When we are in doubt, appeal to principles or policies does not help us decide what to do; yet it is precisely such cases that prompt such appeals in the first place.[15]

This inability to use ethical principles to solve difficult ethical cases results in part from what MacIntyre called the heterogeneity of moral views.[14] MacIntyre asserted that it is precisely because of the lack of consensus about moral theory and ethical analysis that these tools prove to be inadequate in medical ethical dilemmas: "To face issues such as those presented ... is to realize that we have neither the wisdom nor a sort of moral calculus to instruct us on what any set of moral principles may or may not require of us in the concrete, clinical situations of medical practice."[15] Individuals must, therefore, develop what Zaner called a responsive ethic—responsive to clinicians, patients, and families. Such an ethic must meet three requirements:

1. Medical ethics must be well informed about not only medical, but all facts of the case. Moral issues are considered only within the specific context within which they occur.
2. The practice of medicine must be understood in terms of medicine's history, thematic nature, and connection to biomedical science.
3. Medical ethics must be accountable and responsible to providers, patient, and families.[15]

With recent changes in health care delivery, the requirements that medical ethics reflect an understanding of the health care system and accountability to third party payers and the public might also be added to Zaner's requirements.

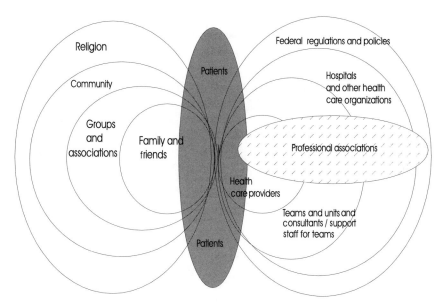

Figure 1.2 Web of social values in which health care occurs. (Adapted from RM Zaner. Ethics and the Clinical Encounter. Englewood Cliffs, NJ: Prentice-Hall, 1988;35.)

To understand the unique context in which health care takes place, Zaner used a phenomenologic analysis of the life world. The patient-provider relationship is one in which both patient and health care provider bring a web of social values influenced by multiple communities of meaning (Figure 1.2). Within this web of values, individuals encounter moral quandaries or conflicts. People deal most easily with problems that are both real and clear, moral problems with which they have experience. On the other hand, individuals have more difficulty with problems that are unanticipated and vague (Figure 1.3). Moral problems encountered outside of the zone of common experience are more difficult to resolve. The difficulty that is experienced in new contexts testifies to the importance of context in ethical decisions.

One important school of medical ethics uses cases to capture the importance of context. Some people refer to this as *casuistry*. Casuistry has deep historical roots in Judaism, Aristotelianism, and common law. In the current landscape, this approach is exemplified by the work of Albert Jonsen and Stephen Toulmin.[16] Jonsen and Toulmin argued that casuistry has been misunderstood, with the consequence that universal principles have been overemphasized. They put forward the following two arguments in favor of the casuistry:

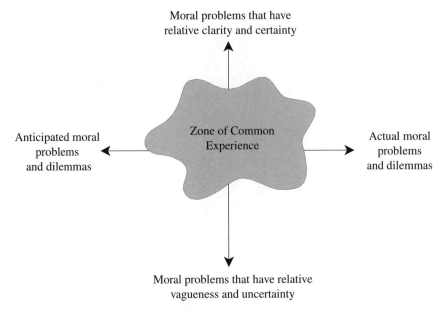

Figure 1.3 Moral problems and the zone of common experience. (Adapted from RM Zaner. Ethics and the Clinical Encounter. Englewood Cliffs, NJ: Prentice-Hall, 1988;44.)

1. The "primary locus of moral understanding" is in the identification of paradigmatic cases of moral conduct. These examples provide a guide for understanding of right or wrong moral conduct.
2. The core of moral knowledge is not in abstract universal propositions but rather in exercising moral discernment relevant to subtle contextual differences.

Although context is an important consideration in ethical decisions, approaches that rely too heavily on context run the risk of being charged with moral relativism. Moral relativists contend that moral judgments are strictly the result of cultural education. Since moral judgments are the product of diverse cultures and customs, it is not possible to make or compare moral judgments across cultures. Extreme moral relativism asserts that moral judgments are not subject to rational analysis and therefore any particular moral judgment is as good as another. Although few people describe themselves as moral relativists, many decry the lack of a moral foundation in current times. In a pluralistic society, it is difficult to distinguish between tolerance for diversity and relativism.

Value

Value, a term frequently used in ethical debates, cuts across all of the categories of ethical analysis. As defined by Harold F. Gortner,[17] "Values ... are standards of desirability, couched in terms of good or bad, beautiful or ugly, pleasant or unpleasant, appropriate or inappropriate that come about, at least in part, through socialization. Beyond the basic values related to survival, individuals develop standards of the desirable through social experience." A society can place value on duties, principles, virtues, or material objects.

Values are formed through the various communities and institutions with which individuals relate during their lives: families, churches, schools, political associations, voluntary associations, national government, and the media. Some of the most deeply held values seem to develop without conscious reflection. For that reason, it can be important to rationally examine values; a process called *values clarification*. Individual and societal values change as a result of dialogue and new experiences. As a result of the civil rights movement, the value of segregation was examined and devalued in favor of the values of justice and equal access.

It is also possible to change the assessment of virtues. During most of history, the virtues of deference and gentleness were valued for women, while men were encouraged to be assertive and decisive. In the Western world, these virtues have been challenged as conflicting with the commitment to equality.

Feminist Ethics and Ethics of Care: Moral Development and Women

Feminist ethics and the ethics of care constitute major alternatives to philosophical approaches to ethics. The philosophical approaches discussed in this chapter's previous sections emphasize abstract principles and rules for behavior. In contrast to philosophical ethics' emphasis on rational evaluation of rules for behavior, moral development addresses the psychological and developmental processes involved in moral behavior. In particular, the ethics of care emphasizes the importance of relationships. Working from the cognitive developmental approach and building on the work of Jean Piaget, Lawrence Kohlberg pioneered theories in the area of learning and internalizing moral concepts and values in 1958.[18] He proposed six stages of moral development[19]:

Stage 1: The morality of obedience: Do what you're told.
Stage 2: The morality of instrumental egoism and exchange: Let's make a deal.

Stage 3: The morality of interpersonal concordance: Be considerate, nice, and kind; you'll make friends.

Stage 4: The morality of law and duty to the social order: Everyone in society is obligated to and protected by the law.

Stage 5: The morality of consensus-building procedures: You are obligated by the arrangements that are agreed to by due process procedures.

Stage 6: The morality of nonarbitrary social cooperation: Morality is defined by how rational and impartial people would ideally organize cooperation.

Although Kohlberg's work emphasized a different aspect of moral behavior, it should be noted that Kohlberg's stages are compatible with the philosophical approach to ethics described in the first part of this chapter. In part, this is because Kohlberg constructed the categories around the concept of justice. Indeed, Kohlberg described his own educational agenda as a developmental-philosophical strategy.[20] One major criticism of Kohlberg's work is that it is overly indebted to rational deontological or universalist philosophers such as Kant, Rawls,[21] and Habermas,[22] particularly in his development of stages 5 and 6.[19]

Another major criticism of Kohlberg's work came from women. Carol Gilligan[23] argued in her book *In a Different Voice* that Kohlberg's stages reflected the experience of men rather than being the universal experience he claimed. While working as a research assistant to Kohlberg, Gilligan noticed that women described their moral experiences very differently than men described theirs. Gilligan[23] and Nel Noddings[24] contended that for women moral development revolved around the concept of care.

> Thus women not only define themselves in a context of human relationship but also judge themselves in terms of their ability to care. Women's place in man's life cycle has been that of nurturer, caretaker, and helpmate, the weaver of those networks of relationships on which she in turn relies. But while women have thus taken care of men, men have, in their theories of psychological development, as in their economic arrangements, tended to assume or devalue that care.[23]

Ironically, it is precisely these "good" qualities of women that result in their lower ranking on Kohlberg's scale. While women see moral dilemmas from the standpoint of relationship and connection, Kohlberg's scale depends on impartiality:

> This different construction of the moral problem by women may be seen as the critical reason for their failure to develop within the constraints of Kohlberg's system. Regarding all constructions of responsibility as evidence of a conventional moral understanding, Kohlberg defines the highest stages of moral development as deriving from a reflective understanding of human

rights. That the morality of rights differs from the morality of responsibility in its emphasis on separation rather than connection, in its consideration of the individual rather than the relationship as primary.[23]

The position of impartiality has important implications for the relationship between provider and patient, as Amy Freedman[25] pointed out. "As applied to the physician-patient relationship, Kantian theory grounds moral judgment on a notion of the physician as an objective, impersonal agent who appeals to universal laws and precludes the discussion of individual context, which is intrinsic to an ethic of care."[25]

Noddings[24] proposed what she and Gilligan called an ethic of care. She located the ontologic starting point for this ethic in human relationships: "An important difference between an ethic of caring and other ethics that give subjectivity its proper place is its foundation in relation."[24] This contrasts with the disinterested, objective perspective of traditional ethics. Noddings also rejected universalizability and founding ethical decisions on principles: "Indeed, I shall reject ethics of principle as ambiguous and unstable. Wherever there is a principle, there is implied its exception and, too often, principles function to separate us from each other."[24]

In the ethics of care, context plays an important role. However, it is not clear how this ethics can inform concrete decisions. Gilligan's work ignited controversies within the fields of ethics in general and medical ethics as well as among feminist thinkers.

Gilligan's critiques and the work of other feminist ethicists illustrate the manner in which some social problems may cut across all categories of analysis. In nursing, it has been argued that preoccupation with autonomy may represent a sexism and that ethics of care may remedy that emphasis. These approaches confirm the need for reflection on the social context and environment in which ethical decisions are made.

Ethical Theories and Approaches

As the analysis of the ethics of care suggests, different ethical theories emphasize different ethical concepts or elements. Although deontological theories emphasize duty, utilitarianism emphasizes consequences, and the ethics of care emphasizes relationships. Table 1.1 summarizes theories of ethics, their bases for ethical decisions, and their proponents.

Summary of Ethical Theories and Categories

It is clear from this overview of ethical theories, categories, and elements that there is no agreement on how to make ethical decisions. It is particularly difficult to derive specific ethical obligations and actions from general moral theories. Because of the lack of agreement about

Table 1.1
Major theories of ethics

Ethical Theory	Basis for Decisions	Representative Thinkers
Deontology	Duty or obligation Kant's categorical imperative	Immanuel Kant[12, 41]
Utilitarianism	Consequences Principle of utility	John Stuart Mill[42] Jeremy Bentham[43]
Character	Virtue or character	Aristotle[44] Edmund Pellegrino[29]
Liberal individualism	Individual rights	John Locke[38] Robert Nozick[39] Ronald Dworkin[40]
Communitarianism	Common good Community or social goals	Alasdair MacIntyre[14] Daniel Callahan[45, 46]
Ethics of care	Relationships	Nel Noddings[24] Much of nursing literature Susan Sherwin[47]
Casuistry	Paradigmatic cases	Stephen Toulmin[16] Albert Jonsen[16]
Principlism (four principles approach)	Principles based in common morality	Tom Beauchamp and James Childress (originators)[27] Dominant model of medical ethics

Source: Adapted from TL Beauchamp, JF Childress. Principles of Biomedical Ethics (4th ed). New York: Oxford University Press, 1994.

the best way to approach ethics, medical ethics has employed the approach of using what might be described as *middle level principles*[26] that address common problems encountered in medicine. This approach, frequently referred to as the *four principles approach*, was popularized by Beauchamp and Childress,[27] who built on the work of Ross. The four principles approach leaves open the question of how to arbitrate conflicting principles. The four principles historically used in medical ethics to generalize the obligations and duties of health care providers are autonomy, beneficence, nonmaleficence, and justice.*

---

*Arras and Steinbock summarized these principles through the following tenets: "In simpler terms, the core principles of bioethics bid us to (1) respect the capacity of individuals to choose their own vision of the good life and act accordingly; (2) foster the interests and happiness of other persons and of society at large; (3) refrain from harming other persons; and (4) act fairly, distribute benefits and burdens in an equitable fashion, and resolve disputes by means of fair procedures."

These principles are the basis for rules of truth-telling, promise-keeping, and confidentiality, all of which presumably honor autonomy, avoid harm, and promote good when they are equitably distributed. The four principles do not exhaust duties, but medical ethicists have used them to describe some of the most common duties. Various ethicists have attempted to determine which duty is primary. For example, Frankena[8] argued that the principle of beneficence embraces nonmaleficence. However, the principle of beneficence does not help in adjudicating conflicts that may arise in distributing good or evil—that is, that the principle of beneficence does not, by itself, assist individuals in determining for whom they ought to promote good. For this, some concept of justice[8] or fairness is needed. Justice refers to equality in the distribution of the good. Distributive justice is concerned with the *"comparative treatment* of individuals."[8]

Principles, Theories, and Rules

It may be useful to consider how theories, principles, and rules are distinguished. Following Beauchamp and Childress, theories, principles, and rules represent increasing levels of specificity with regard to guiding behavior. Ethical theory is the broadest and most general category. An ethical theory encompasses metaethical considerations by specifying how ethical categories relate and what is meant by good and right. In Table 1.1, each theory represents an attempt to delineate the appropriate basis for ethical decisions. Ethical theories do not provide direct guidance as to what should be done in a specific situation. For example, the ethical theory of caring proposes that relationships are the basis of ethical decisions; it does not provide guidance for making these decisions in specific situations.

Principles are more specific than theories in that they provide some guidance for behavior. The principle of beneficence suggests that individuals ought to promote good in their actions. Rules are more specific than either theories or principles. The APTA *Guide for Professional Conduct* contains a number of rules (e.g., therapists are not to accept gifts from patients). Principles and rules may seem to conflict with each other.

DEVELOPMENT OF THE FIELD OF MEDICAL ETHICS

The practice of medicine and the study of ethics have existed since at least the time of the ancient Greeks, but it was not until the 1970s that these two fields came together to produce a new field: medical ethics.

Technologic advances and the increasingly complex institutional setting of medicine produced complex ethical dilemmas.[26, 28] In response
to dilemmas such as the determination of death and decisions about
dialysis, many medical practitioners began to use the tools of the discipline that had historically investigated the nature of right and wrong:
philosophy. The development of the field of medical ethics reflects its
interdisciplinary origins through its use of traditional ethical theories
and principles in moral reasoning about medical situations.

Edmund Pellegrino[29] noted that the dominant paradigm of medical
ethics in the United States has been "principlism." Pellegrino outlined
the four periods in the history of medical ethics as:

1.   The quiescent period, characterized by reliance on the Hippocratic Oath.* The foundation for this ethic was the physician-patient
relationship, but it lacked systematic formalization. According to Pellegrino, the unrest of the 1960s, the demise of shared communal values, loss of trust in institutions, rapid development of technology, and
the depersonalization of health care contributed to the disintegration
of the "Hippocratic synthesis."[29]

2.   The period of principlism (mid-1960s to mid to late 1980s).
Beauchamp and Childress[27] used W.D. Ross's prima facie principles to
develop the four principles approach. The principles blend with the
Hippocratic Oath. Pellegrino[29] noted that autonomy and justice, not a
part of the Hippocratic ethic, were never totally embraced by the medical community.

3.   Antiprinciplism (late 1980s to 1990s). Reaction to weaknesses
of the four principles approach yields three major alternatives: virtue-
based ethics, ethics of care, and casuistry.

4.   Period of crisis (the future). Need for a new philosophical basis
to address moral relativism and postmodernism.

Principlism has been criticized for being abstract, for its inability to
resolve conflicts between competing principles, and for its deductivism.
Deductivism means the application of very abstract principles directly to
specific concrete situations. Deductivism presumes that the correct action
in a particular situation can be derived in a "top-down" fashion from
abstract principles. As Arras and Steinbock[26] suggested, the direct application of very general abstract principles to specific cases is difficult.

These criticisms point to the difficulties encountered by practitioners in applying ethical principles to concrete situations, which often
proves difficult and confusing for the practitioner, due in large mea-

---

*Pellegrino does not provide exact time frames. Time frames were extrapolated from refer-
ences listed.

sure to the fact that principles may conflict. In the case of conflicting principles, there is no clear basis by which to decide between the goals of competing principles. For example, in a case in which a patient arrives late for treatment, the PT must deal with the principles of beneficence (the duty to foster the patient's interests), nonmaleficence (the duty not to harm the patient), and justice (the duty to distribute services equitably),[26] yielding conflicting alternatives. Can others' treatment be justly shortened to promote benefit to the patient who arrived late? The traditional principle-based approach does not by itself provide a way of deciding between conflicting principles.

Another criticism of the traditional principle-based approach to medical ethics is that it ignores the specific and unique context within which medical-ethical decisions are made. For example, the information that the patient has arrived 30 minutes late for each appointment may influence the decision. Or it may be that the facility is operating short-staffed. For just this reason, many have recommended a case-based approach to analyzing these issues.[16] Arras and Steinbock[26] argued that the proper approach to medical ethics is a dialectical or reciprocal use of principles and cases. Rawls[21] described the process of moving between principles and conditions as reflective equilibrium. It is impossible to choose between principles and cases because both are necessary for sound ethical decision making.

PHYSICAL THERAPY AND MEDICAL ETHICS

As a profession, physical therapy has tended to follow the lead of the medical field in using the four principles approach to resolving moral dilemmas. Every new PT is familiar with the ethical principles of autonomy, beneficence, nonmaleficence, and justice, and most have given some thought to the differences between a deontological and a virtue-based or teleological approach to ethics. Ruth Purtilo[11] has been a pioneer in bringing such ethical reflection to the field of physical therapy. Ongoing work will be needed to meet the ethical challenges facing physical therapy in the twenty-first century.

The shortcomings of principle-based, communitarian, case-based, ethics of care, deontological, consequentialist, and virtue-based ethical approaches indicate the current inadequacy of any single approach used to the exclusion of other approaches. This inadequacy points to the need for moral imagination,[30, 31] or the need to emphasize the creative process in solving ethical dilemmas. It is not the case that ethical principles can be applied as mathematical formulations, which yield a single answer to difficult problems. Rather, moral decision making is a

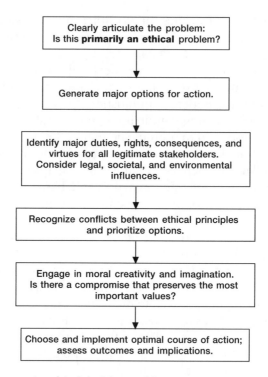

Figure 1.4 Six steps in ethical decision making.

creative process that requires the consideration of traditional principles, virtues, community considerations, specific context, creativity in formulating alternative courses of action, and dialogue with others involved in the problem (moral discourse). Moreover, multiple possible actions may be correct in a particular situation. Traditional approaches have placed far too little emphasis on the role of creativity and imagination and moral discourse in addressing ethical problems.

Decision-Making Process

This text presents a decision-making process that incorporates the traditional principles of ethics, is case based, addresses virtue, acknowledges conflicts between principles, considers consequences, invites consideration of social needs and biases, and advocates moral discourse and creativity. This approach uses and expands the traditional principles approach to ethics but attempts to compensate for some of the shortcomings of that approach by using a case-oriented, decision-making process that addresses weaknesses of the traditional approach.

Figure 1.4 summarizes the six-step decision-making process that is used in this book. The method uses the traditional principle-based approach to ethical dilemmas but supplements it with conscious attention to societal influences and consequences, moral imagination, and the community context of moral discourse. The process is designed to deal with difficult and complex situations that involve a high degree of what Zaner called "moral vagueness and uncertainty."[15] A formal decision-making process is most appropriate for unanticipated and vague moral problems, as illustrated by Figure 1.3.[15] Ethical decisions in situations that are clear and anticipated are easiest, because they require neither clarification nor interpolation in uncharted territory. Frequently, they can be solved through the simple application of a moral principle. These decisions seem to occur almost at a preconscious level. For instance, if a grocery clerk gives a customer too much change, pointing out the mistake and returning the money is a simple case of honesty. There is no real need for a process to sort out conflicting values in such a situation. Indeed, some people would argue that this is not really an *ethical* dilemma because most would agree that the right thing to do is to return the money. The conflict is whether to do the right thing or whether to serve one's immediate financial self-interest. If a large sum of money is involved, this may be a hard choice.[11]

Step 1: Define the Problem

The first step in the six-step approach to decision making is to ask, "Is this primarily an ethical problem that demands analysis?" To decide whether a problem is an ethical one, recall the earlier discussion of the term *ethics*. Based on an understanding of ethics, individuals must decide whether a problem primarily concerns right or wrong human conduct. As previously discussed, the first step of the decision-making process may be very simple if it falls in Zaner's zone of relative certainty. In a very short time, individuals recognize a situation as ethical and determine the correct moral response. Individuals may not always agree on this zone of relative certainty. What may seem to one person to be the exercise of simple morality may be a moral dilemma for someone else because of differing moral, social, religious, or individual contexts. For example, in the simple case previously cited in which the grocery clerk gives the wrong change, suppose that the customer is a member of a poor population that has been systematically price gouged by this store, which enjoys a monopoly in the area. In that case, this situation may no longer fall in the zone of moral certainty. It may now be a dilemma that demands further analysis.

Step 2: Generate Feasible Options

The second step in the decision-making process is to generate no more than three feasible options. *Option* refers to a possible course of action in response to the ethical problem. As in step one, two options may be immediately obvious. In fact, many situations are choices between equally desirable (or undesirable) options. Ruth Purtilo[11] called these situations *ethical dilemmas* and described them as "a common type of problem that involves two (or more) morally correct courses of action *but you can't do both*." In an actual dilemma, taking one course of action may do justice to a particular moral principle or value but prevents doing justice to another.

CASE 1.1

Sarah Giles is a PT who works in a large suburban hospital. Sarah had been treating Mike Peterson for a fractured tibia for 3 weeks when Mike's surgeon took him back to surgery for hardware removal. Sarah learns from an operating room nurse after the surgery that Mike sustained nerve damage through physician error. The nurse asks that she keep this information in confidence. When Mike returns for physical therapy treatment the following week, there is no documentation in the medical record about the error. Mike tells Sarah that he has been wondering if it is normal to have footdrop after hardware removal. He states that he has felt that something went wrong during the surgery. He asks Sarah directly if she knows anything about what happened.

Sarah is faced with an ethical dilemma between the patient's right to know and her promise to keep this information in confidence. (Sarah may also be concerned about the consequences of either action, but that subject is considered under *Law and Ethics*.)

In this case, Sarah has two obvious options: to tell the patient what happened or not to tell the patient. It is appropriate to spend some time at this point making the options specific as a plan. Sarah should think about the specific time, content, and place of her conversation with Mike. Should anyone else be present? She must also determine whether the major options are feasible. At first glance, it seems that both of these options are feasible. However, it is better to think of feasibility in a broader institutional framework. In most hospitals, information from the medical record must come from the medical records department. With the increasing number of alliances and networks, it may also be necessary to investigate beyond the department and the hospital to examine corporate policies.

It is not always so easy to identify two or three major feasible options. It may be necessary to gather more information to formulate some options. For example, Sarah may need to know more about hospital medical records policies or about the law regarding medical records. If Sarah could not identify two or three feasible options, she might seek assistance from a colleague. In seeking help, Sarah must be very careful in selecting someone to talk with, and she should take care to frame her conversations to protect confidential information.

Step 3: Identify Ethical Principles

In the third step of the decision-making process, one must identify ethical principles, recognizing legal, social, contextual, and environmental influences. The worksheet in Figure 1.5 can be used to assist in outlining the pertinent ethical principles. Using the case concerning Sarah Giles, the worksheet might look like Figure 1.6. The major ethical elements have been outlined. If Sarah is unable to identify the major ethical elements, then she should seek the help of a trusted colleague or friend to delineate them.

Sarah might also make use of professional resources, such as the APTA *Guide for Professional Conduct*, to assist her. Sarah should be careful in her selection of a confidant to preserve confidences and to avoid placing the confidant in a difficult ethical situation. For example, Sarah cannot confide in her supervisor until she is prepared for her supervisor to act on behalf of the department's best interests.

Step 4: Prioritize Values Where Conflicts Exist

The next step in the decision-making process is to identify conflicts and prioritize values. Sarah certainly has the ability to tell Mike what she knows. On the worksheet, the duty to disclose has been identified as the most important value. To some extent, prioritization of the values depends on the philosophical orientation of the person making this decision. For example, duty to disclose would be the primary obligation if working from a deontological perspective. A consequentialist or utilitarian might argue that the consequences of telling outweigh the therapist's obligation to disclose this information.

Step 5: Design a Plan

The fifth step in the decision-making process is to design a plan that does justice to competing values and ethical principles.

It seems likely that, in this case, Sarah would place the patient's right to know as a higher priority than loyalty to employer or legal consequences for others. However, it is entirely possible that Sarah may be able to engage in creative problem solving that would yield a plan that satisfies each competing option. For example, Sarah may be able to dis-

Duties, Rights, and Obligations	Anticipated Consequences	Virtues
PT or PTA:		
CLIENT:		

LEGAL, CONTEXTUAL, AND SOCIETAL IMPLICATIONS
LEGAL:
CONTEXTUAL AND ORGANIZATIONAL:
SOCIETAL:

CONFLICTS BETWEEN DUTIES, VIRTUES, CONSEQUENCES, AND CONTEXTUAL OBLIGATIONS

PRIORITY OF VALUES
Can you distinguish prima facie duties from actual duties?

Figure 1.5 Worksheet for outlining ethical principles. (PT = physical therapist; PTA = physical therapist assistant.)

cuss the patient's concerns with the physician. Or Sarah may be able to refer the patient to medical records where the patient would follow appropriate procedures for examining the record. Sarah would also want to involve her supervisor in her decision. Her supervisor may have additional options or may have more authority to negotiate for both patient and therapist. For example, the supervisor may have a close working relationship with the director of the medical records department. In addition, Sarah would not want her supervisor surprised with an unexpected telephone call from an irate physician.

Duties, Rights, and Obligations	Anticipated Consequences	Virtues
PT : 1. Disclose to client relevant information. 2. Keep confidences. 3. Obligation to institution to protect from harm. **CLIENT:** Right to know information regarding health (autonomy).	1. Psychological or physical harm to patient resulting from lack of knowledge. 2. Friend or self may lose job if PT informs patient and patient sues. 3. Possible legal, financial, or professional action against MD.	1. Honesty/truthfulness to patient. 2. Loyalty to friend. 3. Loyalty to MD and institution.

LEGAL, CONTEXTUAL, AND SOCIETAL IMPLICATIONS
LEGAL: Liability of PT, nurse, surgeon, institution for withholding information and for injury to patient. **CONTEXTUAL AND ORGANIZATIONAL:** Ramifications of medical institutions not informing patients of medical information. Erosion of patient rights. Organizational pressures to minimize organizational liability. **SOCIETAL:** Costs of litigious environment of health care.

CONFLICTS BETWEEN DUTIES, VIRTUES, CONSEQUENCES, AND CONTEXTUAL OBLIGATIONS
Duty to disclose to patient and patient's right to know conflicts with duty to keep promise. (Autonomy versus beneficence.) Conflict between the virtues of honesty (toward patient) versus fidelity (toward friend).

PRIORITY OF VALUES
Duty to disclose should take precedence over duty to keep confidences. Moral creativity: How might you act in order to honor both duties?

Figure 1.6 Example of a completed worksheet used to identify ethical issues. (PT = physical therapist; MD = medical doctor.)

Step 6: Choose, Implement, and Reassess Consequences and Social and Environmental Impact

In the final step of the process, Sarah will choose and implement her course of action. She will also reassess the consequences and environmental impact. Suppose that Sarah and her supervisor refer Mike to medical records. At the following treatment session, Mike tells Sarah

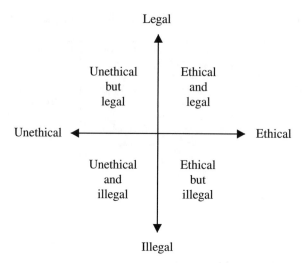

Figure 1.7 Potential relationships between legal and ethical aspects of human behavior.

he has obtained his medical record and shows it to Sarah. In reading the record, Sarah discovers that the surgical report makes no mention of the surgical error. Sarah's priority goal of disclosure has not been accomplished. She must now reassess her options and determine a new course of action.

DISTINCTIONS AND SIMILARITIES AMONG LAW, ETHICS, AND MEDICINE

Law and Ethics

As practicing PTs and administrators know, many clinical situations involve an overlap of legal and ethical issues. Occasionally, legal or ethical issues arise independently, but they often occur in tandem. The best legal solution may not be the best ethical solution in every instance (Figure 1.7).

Laws are usually presumed to reflect a certain level of societal consensus regarding ethical behavior. However, the increasing influence of lobbyists and other special interest groups makes it difficult to assume that laws actually represent majority consensus. In addition, it is questionable whether the United States has a meaningful forum for moral discourse in resolving complex issues, particularly when the matter involves conflicting interests. Although legislatures are supposed to adopt rational policy following reasoned debate, it might be argued that the interests of indi-

Unethical but legal	**Ethical and legal**
Unethical and illegal	**Ethical but illegal**

Figure 1.8 Ethical and legal behavior.

vidual legislators are at times tainted by campaign contributions, lobby-ists, re-election worries, party pressures and other considerations that pre-vent them from carefully examining long-range policy options and implications (see Chapter 7). Another disturbing question is whether all interested parties have a voice in the decision-making process, given the current makeup of federal and state legislatures. Individuals with limited resources may have difficulty making their needs known to those in power. In spite of these reservations, in general, obeying the law is con-sidered the minimal condition for ethical behavior.

Pellegrino[32] described what he called the *ascending order of ethical sensitivity:*

> All professional medical codes, then, are built of a three-tiered system of oblig-ations related to the special roles of physicians in society. In the ascending order of ethical sensitivity they are: observance of the laws of the land, then observance of rights and fulfillment of duties, and finally the practice of virtue.

In Pellegrino's view, to be a virtuous health care provider one must go beyond a legalistic fulfillment of law and duties.

The ascending order of ethical sensitivity implicitly suggests that obeying laws is fundamentally ethical. Indeed, the terms *ethical* and *legal* are frequently lumped together as if they were always identical. That the purpose of a law is to bring about right and good conduct is taken for granted, but it is not always true that legal and ethical actions coincide. In some situations, legal actions seem to be unethical. Pro-viding pro bono services, delivering physical therapy care guided by both law and professional standards, and billing reasonable fees for ser-vices delivered are all both legal and ethical. See Figure 1.8 for a dia-gram of the relationship between these two terms.

In the case of a therapist struggling with reporting suspected abuse, as required by law in some states, the therapist may believe that the eth-

Unethical and illegal	**Ethical and legal**
Unethical and illegal	**Ethical but illegal**

Figure 1.9 Ethical but illegal behavior.

ical demands are in conflict with the legal demands in a specific case. Although the therapist understands the intent of the law, he or she may believe that the patient's interests will be better served by not reporting apparently minor abuse. The therapist may see the situation of the law as conflicting with ethical demands.* A husband who exceeds the speed limit to rush his wife to the hospital to deliver their baby is engaging in illegal activity that most people would regard as ethical. Civil rights activists in the 1960s staged protests in violation of state, local, and federal laws to fulfill ethical demands for justice (Figure 1.9).

There are numerous examples of actions that are both unethical and illegal (see the upper left quadrant of Figure 1.9). Medicare fraud, receiving kickbacks for equipment recommendations, and sexual harassment are unethical and illegal in most states, although there may not necessarily be agreement on how to determine each of these. At times, there appears to be a thin line between legal and illegal. For example, many people stretch their interpretation of tax laws to their advantage. The point at which this process becomes illegal depends on interpretation of the law. A similar process may work in Medicare reimbursement. For example, at what point does the common practice of upcoding diagnoses become unethical or illegal? Unethical actions, both legal and illegal, are represented in Figure 1.10.

Relationship of Law and Ethics to Medicine

The preceding section addressed similarities and distinctions between law and ethics; how do these two disciplines relate to medicine? Much

---

*This is not to say that the therapist is correct in choosing this course of action. Too little information is provided to make that determination. (See Chapter 4 for a discussion of elder and spouse abuse.)

Unethical but legal	Ethical and legal
Unethical and illegal	Ethical but illegal

Figure 1.10 Unethical but legal behavior versus unethical and illegal behavior.

of the work in this area refers primarily to physicians, but many of the principles apply to health care practitioners generally, including PTs. The relationship between medicine and law can be one of conflict. One readily identifiable source of controversy between medical and legal professionals is their varying perceptions of the medical malpractice "crisis" and what, if anything, should be done about it. Additionally, just as medicine has its own jargon, legalese is often imposing and confusing to nonlawyers.

Several commentators suggest that the root of medicolegal differences goes much deeper, however, to the mode of analysis employed by the two disciplines and their corresponding, yet differing, world views.[33–35] One principal difference is the perspective of the two disciplines regarding truth. To health care professionals, truth is a universal, discoverable scientific principle.[33] For lawyers, truth results from opposing points of view aired in a controlled and fair process.

Consider also the question of causation. A physician might indicate a cause of death to be cardiac arrest. A lawyer (or law enforcement officer) looks to the event that is "so closely related to the undesirable end that it ought to give rise to legal liability."[35] Thus, a lawyer may consider the initial gunshot wound that led up to the cardiac arrest as causative. Legal causation tries to represent societal expectations and consensus regarding apportionment of blame.

Another area of distinction between law and medicine is in conflict resolution. Medical tribunals, such as peer review bodies, frequently do not constrain themselves by rules of evidence, such as restrictions on hearsay (often viewed as artificial by health care providers). Such panels are usually composed of experts with knowledge in the area in dispute, as compared to litigation, in which potential jurors are not asked to serve on the jury if they possess prior knowledge of a situation. Lawyers and health care professionals differ as to the relative weight they attach to procedure (or process) and substance.

Health care providers may view their duty to a patient as outweighing their duty to obey the law.[36, 37] For example, a physician may underestimate the age of a fetus in order to provide a therapeutic abortion despite a statutory restriction.

CLINICAL CONTEXT AND THE HEALTH CARE ENVIRONMENT

Several unique aspects of the health care environment—and the PT's clinical context within it—must be understood in considering legal and ethical problems. Health care has traditionally had a relatively hierarchical structure, in which physicians issue orders and PTs (and others) carry them out. With direct access and heightened educational requirements, the nature of physical therapy practice is changing. PTs are more autonomous and use more professional judgment than ever before. Such independence brings more potential legal liability and moral responsibility. Add to this the trend toward delegation within physical therapy services. Hands-on care is often delegated to PT assistants or technicians, with the PT functioning in a supervisory or consultative capacity. Ultimately, however, therapists are legally and morally responsible for all treatment delivered under their supervision (see Chapter 2).

The United States is facing a serious shortage of financial resources and an explosion of costs in the health care arena. Access to health care is a critical problem at the national, state, local, provider, and individual level. Both legal and ethical issues—issues involving right to health care, rationing, and equitable distribution—abound against this backdrop.

A further complicating factor in the American health care system is the method of payment. Those who pay for care (employers, insurers, government entities) are not always the same as those who receive care (patients). The individuals who typically decide what care is needed (providers in concert with patients) may increasingly be overridden by payers. It is often quite difficult for providers to obtain consistent information (regarding precertification, eligibility, etc.) from representatives of third party payers with decision-making authority, although the determinations of these entities often drive provision of care. Add to this the shifting incentives of health care providers from fee-for-service, treatment-oriented plans to capitated plans that encourage less care[25] and the lines of decision making, of legal liability, and of moral responsibility may become blurred.

REFERENCES

1. Health Care Quality Improvement Act of 1986. 42 U.S.C.A. 11101 et seq.
2. *Bryan v. James Holmes Regional Medical Center*, 33 F.3d 1318 (11th Cir. 1994), cert. denied 131 L.E.2d 220 (1995).
3. Tennessee Attorney General Opinion. U94-161 (1994), interpreting Tenn. Code Ann. 63-6-225.
4. Massero TM, O'Brien TL. Constitutional limitations on state-imposed continuing competency requirements for licensed professionals. William & Mary Law Review 1983;25:253.
5. Physician Ownership of, and Referral of Patients or Laboratory Specimens to, Entities Furnishing Clinical Laboratory or Other Health Services, 42 C.F.R. 411.350–.361.
6. Tennessee Rules and Regulations, Physical Therapy—Supervision. 1150-2-.10(2). Board of Occupational and Physical Therapy Examiners (May 1996).
7. Gresham GE, Duncan PW, Stason WB, et al. Post-Stroke Rehabilitation. Clinical Practice Guideline, no. 16. Public Health Service, Agency for Health Care Policy and Research Publication 95-0662. Rockville, MD: U.S. Dept. of Health and Human Services, 1995.
8. Frankena WK. Ethics (2nd ed). Englewood Cliffs, NJ: Prentice-Hall, 1973;4, 6–8, 26, 34–35, 48, 49, 96.
9. Thiroux JP. Ethics: Theory and Practice (5th ed). Englewood Cliffs, NJ: Prentice-Hall, 1995;2, 6, 48, 51, 78.
10. Shaw WH. Social and Personal Ethics. Belmont, CA: Wadsworth, 1993;3, 24, 27–31.
11. Purtilo RB. Ethical Dimensions in the Health Professions (2nd ed). Philadelphia: Saunders, 1993;6, 19, 39.
12. Kant I. On a Supposed Right to Lie from Philanthropy. In MJ Gregor (ed), The Cambridge Edition of the Works of Immanuel Kant: Practical Philosophy. New York: Cambridge University Press, 1996;611–615.
13. Ross WD. The Right and the Good. Oxford, England: Clarendon Press, 1965;19–35.
14. MacIntyre AC. After Virtue (2nd ed). Notre Dame, IN: University of Notre Dame Press, 1984;6–8, 148, 150, 185, 191, 194–195, 236.
15. Zaner RM. Ethics and the Clinical Encounter. Englewood Cliffs, NJ: Prentice-Hall, 1988;16, 26–29, 35, 44.
16. Jonsen AR, Toulmin SE. The Abuse of Casuistry. Berkeley, CA: University of California Press, 1988;330–331.
17. Gortner HF. Values and Ethics. In TL Cooper (ed), Handbook of Administrative Ethics. New York: Marcel Dekker, 1994;378.
18. Rest JR. Development in Judging Moral Issues. Minneapolis: University of Minnesota Press, 1979;7.
19. Rest JR. Background: Theory and Research. In JR Rest, D Narváez (eds), Moral Development in the Professions: Psychology and Applied Ethics. Hillsdale, NJ: Lawrence Erlbaum Associates, 1994;5, 7.
20. Bailey C. Kohlberg on Morality and Feeling. In S Modgil, Celia Modgil (eds), Lawrence Kohlberg: Consensus and Controversy. Philadelphia: Falmer, 1986;197.
21. Rawls J. A Theory of Justice. Cambridge, MA: Belknap Press, 1971.
22. Habermas J. Knowledge and Human Interests. Boston: Beacon Press, 1971.

23. Gilligan C. In a Different Voice: Psychological Theory and Women's Development. Cambridge, MA: Harvard University Press, 1993;17, 19.
24. Noddings N. Caring: A Feminine Approach to Ethics and Moral Education. Berkeley, CA: University of California Press, 1984;5, 6.
25. Freedman A. The physician-patient relationship and the ethic of care. Can Med Assoc J 1993;148:1037–1042.
26. Arras JD, Steinbock B. Ethical Issues in Modern Medicine (4th ed). Mountain View, CA: Mayfield, 1995;34, 35, 37–39.
27. Beauchamp TL, Childress JF. Principles of Biomedical Ethics (4th ed). New York: Oxford University Press, 1994;12, 31–32.
28. Mappes TA, Zembaty JS. Biomedical Ethics (3rd ed). New York: McGraw-Hill 1991;3.
29. Pellegrino ED. The metamorphosis of medical ethics: a 30-year retrospective. JAMA 1993;269:1158–1162.
30. Johnson M. Moral Imagination: Implications of Cognitive Sciences for Ethics. Chicago: University of Chicago Press, 1993.
31. Whitbeck C. Ethics as design: doing justice to moral problems. Hastings Center Report 1996;26:9–16.
32. Pellegrino ED. The Virtuous Physician and the Ethics of Medicine. In EE Shelp (ed), Virtue and Medicine. Dordrecht, Holland: Reidel, 1985;237–255.
33. Gibson J, Schwartz R. Physicians and lawyers: science, art and conflict. Am J Law Med 1980;6:173.
34. Schwartz R. Teaching physicians and lawyers to understand each other. J Legal Med 1981;2:131.
35. Naitove B. Medicolegal education and the crisis in interprofessional relations. Am J Law Med 1982;8:293.
36. Wolf S. Health care reform and the future of physician ethics. Hastings Center Report 1994;24:28–41.
37. Mariner W. Business vs. medical ethics: conflicting standards for managed care. J Law Med Ethics 1995;23:236–246.
38. Locke J. Two Tracts on Government. Cambridge, England: Cambridge University Press, 1967.
39. Nozick R. Anarchy, State, and Utopia. New York: Basic Books, 1974.
40. Dworkin R. Taking Rights Seriously. Cambridge, MA: Harvard University Press, 1977.
41. Kant I. The Metaphysics of Morals. M Gregor (trans and ed). Cambridge, England: Cambridge University Press, 1996.
42. Mill JS. Utilitarianism. In G Williams (ed), On Liberty, Considerations on Representative Government, Remarks on Bentham's Philosophy. Rutland, VT: J.M. Dent, 1993.
43. Bentham J. Deontology Together with a Table of the Springs of Action and the Article on Utilitarianism. New York: Oxford University Press, 1983.
44. Aristotle. The Nichomachen Ethics. JEC Welldon (trans). Amherst, NY: Prometheus Books, 1987.
45. Callahan D. Setting Limits: Medical Goals in an Aging Society. New York: Simon & Schuster, 1987.
46. Callahan D. Allocating health care resources: the vexing case of rehabilitation. Am J Phys Med Rehabil 1993;72:101–105.
47. Sherwin S. No Longer Patient: Feminist Ethics and Health Care. Philadelphia: Temple University Press, 1992.

2

Professional Issues

CASE 2.1

Susan Springer is a physical therapist (PT) employed by Maywood Convalescent Center. At the center, Susan conducts evaluations of patients and supervises treatment provided by two technicians. The center is quite large, and the census is high; Susan is kept busy with clinical and administrative responsibilities. Mrs. Daniels is a 76-year-old woman who underwent a total hip arthroplasty 7 days ago. She spent several days in an acute care facility and has now been transferred to Maywood.

Following her initial evaluation of Mrs. Daniels, Susan establishes an exercise regimen and assigns Mrs. Daniels' treatment to one of the technicians. On her third day at Maywood, Mrs. Daniels arrives in the physical therapy department and tells the technician that she needs to use the bathroom (she has been instructed by the nursing and therapy staff to ask for assistance in using the bathroom). Susan, overhearing the conversation, tells the technician that she needs to remeasure Mrs. Daniels' range of motion and see another patient on the floor; she urges Mrs. Daniels to wait to use the bathroom. After Mrs. Daniels' therapy session, the technician is called to the telephone. Mrs. Daniels stands to walk to the bathroom, but the wheelchair brakes are not locked and she falls, dislocating her hip and fracturing her femur. Mrs. Daniels is returned to the acute care facility for additional surgery; she is hospitalized for 5 days and then transferred to another skilled facility.

What will happen in the event of a lawsuit by Mrs. Daniels against Susan Springer and Maywood?

ELEMENTS OF NEGLIGENCE

The law of medical malpractice usually falls under the law of torts, which involves a personal injury caused by another person.[1]* Malpractice is a form of professional negligence, generally governed by state law. To recover in a negligence case, a plaintiff must prove four elements: (1) that the therapist owed a legal duty to the patient, (2) that the therapist breached that duty, (3) that this breach caused an injury, and (4) that the injury resulted in damages. In most states, plaintiffs must prove the elements—duty, breach, causation, and damages—by a preponderance of the evidence. This means that it is more likely than not that negligence occurred.

Duty

Legal duty is established in the therapy context when there is a patient-therapist relationship. Without a clear relationship, there is no legally imposed duty to come to the aid of another person. For example, a Tennessee court noted that a referring physician is generally not liable for the subsequent negligence of the treating physician.[2] While the law generally imposes no affirmative duty to act, some states have laws that protect individuals who assist in emergency situations in which no underlying relationship exists; these are called *Good Samaritan laws.*[3]

Breach of Duty: Standard of Care

A critical matter in malpractice cases is establishing whether the therapist met the standard of care—that is, did the therapist act in a reasonable manner given the circumstances as compared to what another prudent therapist would do? If not, the standard of care was breached. Depending on the applicable state law, courts apply a national, regional, or locality standard in determining whether the standard of care was met. This is the comparison group against which the therapist's conduct is measured. For example, under the locality rule, the

---

*Some attempts have been made to bring malpractice cases under the law of contracts when a patient contracts with a physician for a particular result (e.g., a certain plastic surgery result). Strict liability theory might also be applied, especially if the matter involves defective equipment. In a rare application of criminal law, a physician was convicted under New York law of reckless endangerment and willful patient neglect for his failure to hospitalize a nursing home patient in a timely manner (*Einaugler v. Supreme Court of State of New York*, 109 F.3d 836 [2nd Cir. 1997]). The patient developed peritonitis and died after the physician mistakenly ordered that feeding solution be administered through her kidney dialysis catheter.

court assesses whether the therapist's conduct is reasonable compared to that of a therapist in the same or similar community. At least one state supreme court that expressly considered the standard of care for PTs concluded that a national standard should apply due to the standardized nature of physical therapy education and training.[4]

In addition to looking at what another reasonable therapist might do under similar circumstances, courts may turn to a variety of other sources to determine the standard of care. These include the scope of practice as defined in the state practice act and the accompanying legislative history, as well as rules adopted by the licensing board. Learned treatises, professional association guidelines, including the American Physical Therapy Association (APTA) *Guide for Professional Conduct*, standards of practice, and clinical practice guidelines or practice parameters can also serve as references.[5] Finally, facility protocols, critical pathways, and policies and procedures can all serve as evidence of what another reasonable therapist would do under such circumstances.*

Causation and Harm

One of the issues contested most often in negligence cases is causation. If the therapist owed a duty to the patient and acted outside the standard of care, the plaintiff must still show that the actions of the therapist caused the injury. If the patient cannot show a causal link between the injury and the action of the therapist, the patient cannot recover damages. In rare cases, the plaintiff can show that there must have been negligence on the part of the therapist; otherwise, the injury could not have occurred. This is known as the doctrine of *res ipsa loquitur*, or "the thing speaks for itself." An example in the medical context is the case of an individual who sustained a shoulder injury during an appendectomy, presumably due to negligent positioning.[6]

One case that highlights the issue of causation is *St. Paul Fire and Marine Insurance Company v. Prothro*.[7] In this case, a patient alleged that he had acquired a staphylococcus infection resulting from a fall in the physical therapy Hubbard tank that reopened his total hip replacement surgical site. The appellate court found that the issue of causation was appropriate for jury determination—that is, the jury was to decide whether the fall caused the infection. A subset of causation is foreseeability. The injury must have been foreseeable and, thus, preventable by the therapist. Harm is also a necessary element. Even if a therapist acted negligently and outside the standard of care, the plaintiff cannot recover if there was no injury.

---

*Note that facility protocols may exceed legal or other recognized standards and establish a higher standard of care.

Who Is to Blame?

Contributory and Comparative Negligence

States have wrestled with several mechanisms for apportioning blame and damages when more than one party is at fault in a negligence action. Under one theory of negligence, if the plaintiff is at all responsible for the injury, he or she is not entitled to collect damages. This is called *contributory negligence* and was the law at one time in many states. Many states have now adopted comparative negligence theory; under this system, if both parties are at fault, their relative contribution to the injury is determined and the damages apportioned accordingly. This issue arose in the case of *Gilles v. Rehabilitation Institute of Oregon*[8] in which a jury was asked to decide whether the plaintiff (a patient status post total hip arthroplasty) was guilty of contributory negligence by grabbing a handrail on a tilt table, pulling herself downward, and refusing to let go while the table was being lowered.

Respondeat Superior and Corporate Negligence

An employer is responsible for the acts of its employees under the doctrine of respondeat superior. Under this theory, liability is imposed on the facility if an employee is negligent while performing duties within the scope of employment. The facility is not liable for the actions of a nonemployee, such as an independent contractor. Thus, a hospital was found not liable for the acts of a transcutaneous electrical nerve stimulation unit distributor who conducted an unauthorized vaginal examination of a hospitalized patient.[9] Even if the individual is clearly employed by the hospital, the employee must be performing duties within the scope of employment—that is, duties on behalf of the employer. The scope-of-employment issue has been raised in several sexual misconduct cases, in which employers have argued that acts undertaken for an employee's sexual gratification should not be treated as falling within the scope of employment.* (See the discussion of sexual misconduct in Chapter 4.)

The corporate negligence doctrine requires that health care facilities provide suitable trained staff, facilities, and policies to provide patients with adequate care. In a seminal case, a hospital was found liable for

---

*Courts have split in this area. Compare, for example, *Samuels v. Southern Baptist Hospital,* 594 So.2d 571 (La. App. 4th Cir.), *app. denied,* 599 So.2d 316 (1992), in which the hospital was found vicariously liable for sexual assault by a nursing assistant on a 16-year-old patient in a psychiatric unit, with *Taylor v. Doctors Hospital,* 21 Ohio App. 3d 154, 486 N.E. 2d 1249 (1985), in which sexual assault by an orderly was found not to be within the scope of employment.

damages sustained by a young patient with a femur fracture who developed gangrene, resulting in an amputation.[10] Issues submitted to the jury in this case were that the hospital (1) failed to provide a sufficient number of trained nurses for bedside care capable of recognizing the progressive gangrenous condition of the plaintiff's leg and of alerting the hospital administration and medical staff so that adequate consultation and treatment could have been provided, (2) failed to require consultation with or examination by hospital surgical staff skilled in such treatment, and (3) failed to review treatment rendered and require consultants as needed.

Application to Case 2.1

For Mrs. Daniels to be successful in a suit against Susan and Maywood, the four elements of negligence—duty, breach, causation, and damages—must be present.

Clearly, Susan and the center owe a duty to Mrs. Daniels; she is a patient in the facility and is receiving physical therapy care under Susan's direct supervision. Failure to permit Mrs. Daniels to use the bathroom before therapy and failure to lock the wheelchair brakes may well have breached the standard of care. This would be a fact question for a jury to decide. (See *Zucker v. Axelrod*,[11] in which a PT was disciplined for failing to permit an elderly nursing home resident to use the bathroom before therapy.)

Causation appears relatively clear, also, but is again a fact question for the jury. Was the hip unstable before the fall? Foreseeability may be an issue; could Susan foresee that Mrs. Daniels might attempt to stand? Was she on a diuretic or did she have a urinary tract infection? (See Chapter 5 for a discussion of foreseeability in fall cases.) Had Mrs. Daniels been assisted to the bathroom earlier, she may not have attempted to stand independently; had the brakes been locked, she may not have fallen. Finally, there do appear to be clear damages arising from the incident. Mrs. Daniels had to undergo additional surgery and hospitalization as well as pain and suffering; the related expenses likely are compensable damages.

The outcome will be affected by state law. If the incident occurred in a state that recognizes contributory negligence, Mrs. Daniels may not be successful because she stood up despite clear instructions that she should request assistance, presuming she is mentally capable of following such instructions. If the state applies a comparative negligence theory, the damages may be apportioned between the parties.

Will Maywood be liable for Susan's actions? Recall that an employer is responsible for the acts of its employees acting within the scope of employment. Health care facilities must also provide suitable trained staff, facilities, and policies to provide patients with adequate care under corporate negligence theory. As both Susan and the technician were Maywood employees acting within the scope of their duties, a court could impose liability on Maywood under the doctrine of respondeat superior.

Suppose Susan was not an employee of Maywood but rather was a contract therapist with her own liability insurance. In that case, the facility would likely be liable for the portion of Mrs. Daniels' injuries attributable to the technician, if any. If Mrs. Daniels can show that the facility was negligent in its policies and procedures, staff training, or physical facilities, liability could also be imposed as corporate negligence.

Note that prevention of another similar situation is critical for the institution. Risk management principles (discussed in Chapter 4) would suggest that all employees be made aware of patient rights and responsibilities and that good communication skills be stressed. "The top 5 reasons for suits against physical therapists relate to communication and the understanding or lack of understanding that can result."[12] These include lack of rapport between the physical therapist and patient or family member, between patient and office staff, unmet patient expectations, and collection activities. Adequate communication and respect for patient needs may well have prevented a lawsuit by Mrs. Daniels.

ETHICAL ANALYSIS

It is often the case that ethical duties and obligations exceed legal duties, which is well illustrated by Case 2.1. It was noted that, from a legal standpoint, Susan may be found negligent if it can be proved that she failed to fulfill her legal duties to Mrs. Daniels. Susan Springer had a legal duty to Mrs. Daniels based on the patient-therapist relationship, but she also had professional duties based on that relationship.

In this case, the decision-making process will not be followed step by step because the case is being dealt with retrospectively and without a dilemma on which to focus. The pertinent ethical questions raised by this case are

1. What were Susan Springer's professional obligations (duties) to the patient?
2. In what ways did Susan Springer fulfill or fail to fulfill her professional obligations to Mrs. Daniels?

3. What contextual pressures worked to create this ethical problem?

4. What actions can a PT take to avoid such outcomes?

Duties, Rights, and Obligations: Autonomy versus Beneficence and Nonmaleficence

Case 2.1 presents itself as a therapist's attempt to balance autonomy and beneficence. Specifically, Susan was balancing Mrs. Daniels' needs for self-determination in going to the restroom and the clinical desire to provide efficient care. The provision of efficient care is broadly interpreted here as a kind of beneficence.

The ethical principles of beneficence and nonmaleficence emphasize the duties of the provider to promote good (beneficence) while avoiding harm (nonmaleficence) through his or her actions. The APTA *Code of Ethics* and *Guide for Professional Conduct* include injunctions toward beneficence, nonmaleficence, and respect for autonomy. The *Code* emphasizes respect for the "rights and dignity of all individuals" and the *Guide* elaborates on that principle as being guided by the patient's "physical, psychological, and socioeconomic welfare."

The term *beneficence* derives from the Latin terms *bene* (well) and *facere* (to do).[13] To do the right thing from the standpoint of the principle of beneficence involves the following three components, as defined by Jacques Thiroux[14]:

1. Promote goodness over badness and do good (beneficence).
2. Cause no harm or badness (nonmaleficence).
3. Prevent badness or harm (nonmaleficence).

Like most writers in this area, Thiroux linked beneficence with nonmaleficence. The problem is that in promoting one good, some harm may be caused. The Catholic doctrine of the double effect recognizes that even good actions can produce both good and bad effects.[15] The Hippocratic Oath placed the prevention of harm as the starting point of medicine: "Primum nocere," or "first, do no harm."

The fundamental duty of beneficence within this context was to promote Mrs. Daniels' health and prevent injury to her. Did Susan fulfill her obligation to prevent injury to Mrs. Daniels? By placing Mrs. Daniels in a situation in which she was unable to attend to her needs safely, it would seem that Susan failed to fulfill her duties of beneficence and nonmaleficence.

Indirectly Susan may have further failed in her obligations by failing to adequately train and supervise the technician to prevent harm to the patient. An implicit suggestion of the APTA *Guide for Professional Conduct* (Principle 3) is that PTs have an obligation to create reliable systems to train support personnel. Had the technician been properly trained in safety matters, such as locking the wheelchair brakes? Had the technician been properly trained to report back to the therapist concerning Mrs. Daniels' urgent need to go to the bathroom?

In Chapter 1, the logical connection between rights and duties was discussed. In part, obligations can be said to flow from an individual's sense of existing rights. Susan's professional duties and obligations to Mrs. Daniels issue in part from Mrs. Daniels' right to dignity and autonomy—that is, if Mrs. Daniels had a right to autonomy, then Susan had some obligation to fulfill that right if she were able to. Specifically, in this case, it is obvious that Mrs. Daniels had a right to autonomy with regard to using the bathroom. Insofar as Susan was able to assist Mrs. Daniels with fulfilling this function, she had an obligation to do so. Clearly, Mrs. Daniels' right to autonomy and dignity were compromised in this situation.

Although this case deals with a fairly straightforward scenario, it is often difficult to reach agreement on cases involving autonomy. It is clear that autonomy can mean different things in various contexts when individual protection is at stake. Autonomy for a child playing near a street may mean something totally different from autonomy for an adult with advanced multiple sclerosis. Because the notion of autonomy plays such a major role in medical ethics, a further explication of the meaning of autonomy is helpful.

Bruce Miller[16] identified what he called *four senses of autonomy*.

> At the first level of analysis it is enough to say that autonomy is self-determination, that the right to autonomy is the right to make one's own choices, and that respect for autonomy is the obligation not to interfere with the choice of another and to treat another as a being capable of choosing. This is helpful, but the concept has more than one meaning. There are at least four senses of the concept as it used in medical ethics: autonomy as free action, autonomy as authenticity, autonomy as effective deliberation, and autonomy as moral reflection.

When autonomy is referred to as free action, the primary dimensions of being voluntary and intentional are identified.[16] These conditions are not always easy to determine when patients are either mentally compromised or under extreme duress. At least in theory, the doctrine of informed consent addresses autonomy as free action. While granting consent to be treated addresses the dimension of voluntariness, disclosure of information addresses the dimension of intentionality. (See Chapter 6 for a discussion of informed consent.)

The second sense in which autonomy is used is in the sense of authenticity. "Autonomy as authenticity means that an action is consistent with the person's attitudes, values, dispositions, and plans. Roughly, the person is acting in character."[15] Autonomy in the sense of authenticity may be difficult to determine in the medical context. Patients are in an unfamiliar setting, undergoing stressful procedures. Little may be known of the patient's character outside of the medical environment. It may not be possible to determine authenticity in most situations, and it may not normally be important to know. However, examining the authenticity sense of autonomy can help in making critical decisions, such as continuing life-support. Families may say, "Mother would not want to continue to live like this."

To be an autonomous decision, the decision must reflect effective deliberation.[16] Effective deliberation indicates that the patient understands the options and ramifications of the situation and has chosen a course of action after due consideration. In brief, the decision is not merely an impulse based on whim or temporary circumstance.

Autonomy as moral reflection indicates a patient's examination of and acceptance of the moral values on which his or her action is based. This sense of autonomy may be difficult to assess, as individuals possess various levels of interest in or ability to engage in this sort of reflection.

The four senses of autonomy, as described by Miller, are related to each other, with free action the foundation for all other senses of autonomy.

> It is important to note that if the action is not a free action then it makes no sense to assert *or* deny that the action was autonomous in any of the other senses. A coerced action cannot be one that was chosen in accord with the person's character and life plan, nor one that was chosen after effective deliberation, nor one that was chosen in accord with moral standards that the patient has reflected upon. The point is the same if the action is not intentional.[16]

Miller's distinctions may be helpful when attempting to sort through a complex situation in which someone has requested to forego further treatment. However, few people's everyday actions qualify as autonomous by Miller's criteria. By establishing such ideal standards for autonomy, the concept is removed from the realm of common experience.[17]

The concept of autonomy has played an important role in the development of the liberal democratic tradition. In fact, some people argue, as Alasdair MacIntyre[18] did, that autonomy has been over-emphasized in ethical and social deliberations in our culture. In a society of autonomous individuals acting only on self-interest, it is not possible to achieve consensus on social matters, a point that MacIntyre fully elaborated.

No person can have complete autonomy. Living in relationship to others involves trade-offs with loss of self-determination. Moreover, in different societies, people are permitted different degrees of autonomy.

Voluntarily entering the health care delivery system represents a decision to relinquish some control over self-determination (decisions about autonomy are even more difficult in emergency situations, when the patient is unable to act autonomously due to the extent of injury). Debate frequently centers around determination of appropriate levels of autonomy for individuals whose judgment may be compromised or not fully developed. Typically, the ethical debate around these conflicts is framed as a conflict between autonomy and beneficence. For example, following traumatic brain injury, a person may have the desire to live independently but may actually lack appropriate judgment to do so. In such a situation, there may be perceived conflict between the principles of autonomy and beneficence. If the patient is granted total self-determination, his or her best interests may not be promoted because he or she is not being protected from harm. The ethical challenge is to determine what level of autonomy is appropriate and possible and to establish a process that safeguards individual rights.

Autonomy and Rehabilitation

Bruce Jennings[19] noted that the concept of autonomy may be inadequate for analyzing the ethical dilemmas of rehabilitation. The rehabilitation context demands some notion of the "good life" in relation to the patient's future prospects. "What is important here is the fact that some such interpretation of the meaning of the patient's future prospects (some construal of the good life to which the patient can and should be restored) is an integral part of the patient/provider/family relationship in rehabilitation."[19]

According to Jennings, traditional individualistic notions of autonomy are inadequate to the collaborative task of rehabilitation. Jennings describes the dilemma as follows:

> Every moral instinct in our liberal, pluralist society tells us that all competent adults should be able to define their own good in the their own way. At the same time, both the medical and social realities of rehabilitation (and other forms of long-term care) belie this atomistic picture of individual self-fashioning and self-sovereignty. Meaning comes through relationships, empowerment through dependency, and the goal is not to shape circumstances but to be shaped by unchosen circumstances in the most affirming way feasible. Only through therapeutic and care-giving relationships of a special type can the patient's good be mutually discovered rather than unilaterally imposed by another. Only in that way can one walk the line between a demeaning and manipulative professional paternalism, on the one hand, and a romantic, but clinically, and even humanly unreal, ideal of autonomy on the other.[19]

Jennings concluded by noting that the bioethics vocabulary available to rehabilitation is inadequate to this task.

Consequences and Intentions

The *Guide for Professional Conduct* (Principle 3) states that PTs have an obligation to exercise sound judgment. Retrospectively, it is easy to conclude that Susan failed to exercise sound judgment by asking Mrs. Daniels to wait without establishing Mrs. Daniels' ability to do so. The consequence of failing to exercise sound judgment in this case was loss of autonomy and dignity and, ultimately, personal injury for Mrs. Daniels. In ethical as well as legal analysis, it must be asked: Could Susan have anticipated that asking Mrs. Daniels to postpone her trip to the bathroom would result in a fall? Undoubtedly Susan would not have acted in this manner had she known with certainty the consequence of her action; it was not her intention to harm Mrs. Daniels. In the end, Susan's ethical behavior cannot be judged on the basis of intention or unintended consequences.

Context: Mitigating Circumstances?

Although it is quite clear that Susan Springer failed in her ethical obligations in this situation, it is not difficult to appreciate the pressures that may have influenced her decisions. It may be helpful to reflect on how this situation may have evolved for Susan. As discussed in Chapter 1, the medical environment is a complex one requiring the ability to juggle numerous schedules concurrently and direct patient care through the use of support personnel. Case 2.1 suggests that Susan was carrying a heavy load of patients. At any one time, Susan may be responsible for the simultaneous care of four patients. To provide care for everyone, Susan knows she must carefully orchestrate the care of her patients. If Mrs. Daniels spends 20 minutes in the bathroom, Susan will be 20 minutes behind for each subsequent patient. Susan may have conceptualized the situation as a matter of both practicality and justice. Or she may have worked from a utilitarian viewpoint in attempting to bring about the greatest good for the greatest number. She may have reasoned that it would be unjust for everyone to wait because Mrs. Daniels needed to go to the bathroom. Suppose that Mrs. Daniels requested to use the bathroom at every treatment session as a way to avoid rehabilitation. The situation may also be interpreted as Susan balancing time efficiency, justice for other patients, and Mrs. Daniels' rights and needs. In retrospect, it is obvious that Mrs. Daniels' right to autonomy and dignity should have more value than the needs of efficiency, but that is because the consequences of Susan's actions are known. It is unlikely that Susan anticipated this outcome. Viewed as an example of operating from the utilitarian viewpoint, this case demonstrates the difficulty of protecting individual rights from this perspective.

Although it may be agreed that Susan was operating within a high-pressure work environment, Susan did fail to prevent harm to her patient and compromised her patient's right to dignity, and her patient sustained an injury while acting to restore her dignity and meet her own needs.

Moral Imagination: Proactive Moral Action

It is easy to analyze consequences retrospectively, but considerably more difficult to anticipate consequences in advance. What actions must PTs take to prevent these situations from arising? The challenge is to create institutional structures that embody the values, rights, and goals of beneficence that the APTA *Code* and *Guide* describe. What steps can be taken to build humane and responsive organizations that also operate efficiently? This case emphasizes the need to adequately train support personnel to deal with patients and clients. Had the technician recognized that Mrs. Daniels was unable to postpone her trip to the bathroom, he or she might have simply attended to this problem and notified Susan. In addition, PTs have an obligation to analyze their workload. If Susan had more responsibilities than she could fulfill, how might she approach her employer?

QUESTIONS AND NOTES FOR FURTHER REFLECTION

1. Which portions of the professional guides are most helpful in analyzing Case 2.1?

2. How should training programs be designed to develop ethical behaviors and sound judgment among those we supervise?

3. What types of staffing patterns are most conducive to the goals of efficiency, safety, and ethical physical therapy services? What kind of safeguards should we have to prevent adverse outcomes? What legal and ethical topics should be included in training technicians?

4. Has Susan violated the duties described in the *Code of Ethics* and *Guide for Professional Conduct*? (See Chapter 3 for a discussion of the judicial process.)

5. What kind of process should be used when considering limiting a patient's autonomy?

6. What is the obligation to limit autonomy when the consequences of a patient's exercise of autonomy will produce injury? (See Chapter 5.)

7. Note that, in Case 2.1, if a damage award is paid to Mrs. Daniels or even if she receives an amount in settlement of the case, the award or settlement must be reported to the National Practitioner Data Bank.

8. Which standard do you believe ought to apply to PTs: a local, regional, or national standard? Does this standard work well for all types of physical therapy settings? For all experience levels?

9. What are the implications of practice parameters for professional liability in malpractice cases?

10. What steps could Maywood take to prevent this type of injury (and subsequent lawsuit) in the future? (See Chapter 4 for a discussion of risk management principles.)

LIABILITY INSURANCE

The Springer case illustrates the interplay of institutional factors and professional judgment that may come together to produce an adverse outcome for a patient. As accidents do occur, therapists need to be prepared for unforeseen circumstances such as this, typically through liability insurance. An individual's decision whether to purchase liability insurance may depend on the setting in which he or she practices. Health care facilities usually provide insurance to employee health care professionals, but job applicants should inquire about insurance coverage during the interview process, especially if part-time employment is anticipated. Individuals who are functioning as independent contractors rather than employees and who are not covered by the facility's policy should be covered by some form of liability insurance.

As indicated, direct access, evaluate-and-treat orders, postbaccalaureate professional education, private practice, and direct billing all point to heightened responsibility and, therefore, potential liability. Exposure can depend on practice setting. Therapists functioning in private practice and home care might choose to seek additional coverage due to their greater autonomy. Liability insurance may also be more advisable for supervisors, who may be held responsible for the actions of subordinates.

All professional actions, such as peer review, consulting, wellness screening, and supervision, should be delineated. The therapist should understand whether the policy covers licensure actions and civil suits. In addition, exclusions (i.e., for sexual misconduct or criminal liability) should be clarified.

Once a decision is made to obtain insurance coverage, the therapist must understand the limitations of the policy being purchased. There are two primary types of policies—claims made and occurrence. Claims-made policies cover only those claims made or reported during the policy year. Occurrence policies cover all incidents arising during a policy year, regardless of when they are reported to the insurer.

A facility claims-made policy typically covers a therapist only while he or she is employed at the facility and does not cover the therapist once the employment relationship ends. Therapists may obtain extended reporting ("tail") coverage from a prior carrier for incidents that took place during the policy period but were not reported before policy expiration. Prior acts ("nose") coverage covers actions that took place but were not reported before a policy's effective date and is obtained from a new carrier.

Where Do We Stand? Incidence and Trends

Precise incidence tracking is difficult with respect to medical malpractice and is beyond the scope of this work. The question is complex: Do we assess claims filed with insurance companies, lawsuits initiated, judgments awarded, or malpractice premiums in ascertaining whether the malpractice system is escalating into crisis? In addition, one must closely scrutinize research in this area due to the highly political nature of the subject.

The American Medical Association[20] lists the number of malpractice claims as follows:

1985, 10 claims per 100 physicians
1988, 6.4 claims per 100 physicians
1989, 7.4 claims per 100 physicians
1990, 7.7 claims per 100 physicians

During this period, the average award in medical malpractice cases was:

1985, $1,179,095
1989, $1,109,660

Of interest in comparison is the number of injuries caused by health care practitioners. The Harvard Medical Malpractice Study Group[21] conducted an extensive review of medical records of more than 30,000 patients. The group estimated that more than 150,000 iatrogenic fatalities occur annually and that more than half are due to negligence. According to the study, only 1 in 8 injured persons files a claim and 1 in 16 injured persons is compensated.

It has been reported that Citizen Action, a consumer advocacy group, found that average physician premiums for malpractice insurance have dropped 20% since 1988 and that malpractice lawsuits have dropped 23% since 1985.[22] Paul Weiler,[23] a principal member of the Harvard Medical Malpractice Study Group, reported that premiums for medical malpractice insurance rose from $500 million to $1 billion from 1974 to 1976, to $2.5 billion in 1983, and to an astounding $7 billion in 1988. He noted, however, that malpractice premiums for most physicians represent a relatively minor component of their total expenses and that during the 1980s doctors on average preserved their real net income position through a rise in the cost to patients.

In another study reviewing 197,230 claims reported from 182 liability carriers, losses for physiatry were similar to low-risk category specialties such as pathology and psychiatry.[24] One-fourth of the successful claims (and one-third of the dollar losses) were associated with physical therapy. Cases involving femoral fracture comprised 14% of paid claims, with other significant claims for conditions of the vertebral column and medication error.

Physical therapy malpractice claims are relatively rare compared to claims against physicians; the exact number of claims, however, is difficult to obtain. Tracking by one private insurer showed an average claim frequency rate of 0.51% from 1983 to 1987.[25] A study by the U.S. Department of Health and Human Services, as reported by Scott,[25] showed a claim frequency of 1.2% from 1981 to 1986. However, he noted that claims frequency rates appeared to be rising; during several years before 1989, the rate rose 13% per year, according to the APTA's director of insurance and business services. In addition, Ron Scott[26] suggested that the number of reported cases in physical therapy appears to be rising, noting that 27 cases of physical therapy malpractice were reported from 1960 through April 1996, eight of which were tried after 1990.

What types of suits are common in physical therapy? According to one insurance company, the most common complaints involve slips and falls, including falls in whirlpools, and burns from hot packs.[27] The APTA-sponsored insurance program lists as most frequent causes of claims (1) failure to treat properly, including therapeutic exercise and modalities; and (2) failure to refer. Examples include burns, reinjury, unnecessary care, and sexual misconduct.[12] Other causes of physical therapy claims include

- Fractures during passive stretching
- Injuries associated with malfunction of traction machine
- Hip dislocation during range-of-motion exercises following total hip arthroplasty
- Lack of informed consent
- Failure to obtain desired results[28]

Is the System Working? Tort Reform

Tort reform is the response of many states to an outcry from the health care industry, largely from physicians perceiving that medical malpractice litigation poses a crisis for their practices. A variety of approaches have been taken at the state level, including

- Caps on damages awards
- Alternative dispute resolution forums, including mediation and arbitration
- Shortened statutes of limitation (the length of time that a patient has to file suit following the injury)
- Strict regulation of insurance practices
- Limited discovery periods
- Penalties imposed against plaintiffs filing frivolous claims
- Certificate of expert witness that claim has merit
- Limited contingency fees (percentage to lawyer decreases as award to plaintiff increases)
- Abrogation of collateral source rule (damages limited to costs not paid by social security benefits, employer's insurance company, or any other source except family assets)
- Structured awards such as periodic payments or establishment of a trust fund[29]

New initiatives have also been considered at the federal level, including caps on damage awards. The 1997 federal budget proposal contained a $250,000 cap on punitive damages for medical malpractice cases.[30]

National Practitioner Data Bank

The National Practitioner Data Bank is a national computerized repository for information about adverse actions and medical malpractice payments. It was created by the Health Care Quality Improvement Act and became operational September 1, 1990.[31]

Any entity making a payment "in settlement of or in satisfaction in whole or in part of a malpractice claim or judgment against [a] physician, dentist, or other health care practitioner for medical malpractice" must report the payment to the data bank within 30 days of making the payment.[32] Information contained in the data bank regarding medical malpractice payments "shall not be construed as creating a presumption that medical malpractice has occurred."[33] Information in the data bank regarding medical malpractice payments

- Applies to payments based on medical malpractice claims only
- Includes reports of settlements

- Applies to all health care practitioners, not just physicians
- Includes reports of all payments, no matter how small (this has been an ongoing area of controversy, due to the common practice of settling small "nuisance suits")

Confidentiality language within a settlement agreement does not relieve the payer of the duty to report to the data bank.

The data bank also contains information about disciplinary actions taken by state boards and by professional societies against their licensees or members. Currently, this is only required for physicians and dentists and is voluntary for other professionals. The law contemplates addition of other health care professionals, but this measure has been placed on hold due to funding considerations and the logistics of information management.

Who can gain access to information in the data bank? All hospitals must query the data bank when an individual initially applies for staff privileges and every 2 years thereafter.[34] The requirement applies with respect to all physicians, dentists, and other health care practitioners with clinical privileges, including courtesy privileges and "moonlighting" residents. Hospitals that fail to query are considered to have knowledge of all information in the data bank at the time of the mandated query. All other queries are voluntary. Individuals and institutions permitted to query the data bank include

- Health care entities that are entering or considering employment of or affiliation relationships with a physician, dentist, or health care practitioner
- Individuals, who may query the data bank about themselves
- Boards of medical examiners
- Hospitals, with respect to members of the medical staff
- Health care entities, with respect to professional review activity
- Persons seeking data without identifying information
- An attorney or individual who has filed a medical malpractice action requesting information about an individual named in the claim (information is disclosed only with evidence that the hospital failed to query data bank as required)

In the first 19 months of its operation, the data bank processed 33,442 total reports, of which 28,186 were reports of medical malpractice payments.[35] Of the malpractice payments, 2,988, or 10.6%, involved health care practitioners other than physicians and dentists (payments made on behalf of PTs are not specifically broken out). From September 1990 through December 1993, hospitals filed reports on 3,154 practitioners regarding adverse actions. It is unclear whether this low reporting rate reflects improved quality efforts or a tendency for hospitals to not impose suspensions greater than 30 days because of the reporting requirement.[36]

Massachusetts has launched its own version of the National Practitioner Data Bank.[37] Information regarding physician credentials, licensure, and medical malpractice actions is available to the public. Initial reports suggest that the data bank has been fielding large numbers of information requests. Arkansas requires, under the Physical Therapy Practice Act, that PTs and physical therapist assistants (PTAs) notify the state board of physical therapy within 10 days of receipt of notification of a malpractice claim.[38]

CASE 2.2

Laura Edwards is a newly hired PT on her first job. Three months after she is hired, another new PT, Bob Smith, receives word that he has failed the licensing examination. Under the state practice act, he must surrender his temporary license. Their supervisor asks Laura to meet with her and with Bob. She proposes that Bob continue to evaluate and treat patients and that Laura cosign his notes. What are the legal and ethical ramifications of this situation?

This situation presents a dilemma. In Chapter 1, a decision-making process for working through possible ethical dilemmas was described. Following is an example of how those decision-making steps may be used to analyze Laura's situation.

Step 1: Define the problem   Is this an ethical problem? Because the dilemma deals with whether cosigning notes is right or wrong morally, this is an ethical problem.

Step 2: Generate feasible options   Two obvious options present themselves in this case. Laura can either agree to cosign Bob Smith's notes or not agree to cosign the notes.

Step 3: Identify ethical principles   Laura's major duties are

- Her duty to society to practice within the boundaries of the state practice act. This duty is captured by Principle 2 of the *Guide for Professional Conduct*: "Physical therapists comply with the laws and regulations governing the practice of physical therapy."
- Her duty to her employer to provide care for patients.
- Her duty to patients to provide appropriate, safe, and legal care. This is captured by Principle 7 of the *Guide*: "Physical therapists accept the responsibility to protect the public and the profession from unethical, incompetent, or illegal acts." Another dimension of this duty is elaborated in Principle 3.2A:

"Physical therapists shall not delegate to a less-qualified person any activity which requires the unique skill, knowledge, and judgment of the physical therapist."

The major right involved is the patients' right to safe treatment administered by a qualified PT. The major virtues would include

- Laura's loyalty to her employer and coworker (would it make a difference if Bob were Laura's close friend?)
- Veracity in representation of services to public and patients
- Accountability to consumers and public

The possible consequences are

- Possible adverse or professional consequences for participation in misrepresentation of services (in most states, Bob is now viewed as a technician; a technician, therefore, is now evaluating and treating patients).
- If Laura refuses to cosign the notes, her employer may have to fire Bob (her employer may not be able to afford to pay a therapist's salary to a person who is functioning as a technician).
- Possible injury to a patient for whom Laura is legally and professionally responsible. (Although it might be assumed that Bob, a graduate of an accredited program of physical therapy, is qualified to be a PT and will eventually pass the examination, objectively until Bob passes he is not qualified to practice as a PT. If a patient were to be injured by Bob, the claim might be made that Laura was morally and professionally culpable for allowing someone to treat who was known to be unqualified.)
- If the clinic is understaffed, it may be difficult for patients to be seen. Some patients who need physical therapy may not receive it.

These duties and rights can also be described in terms of the principles of beneficence and nonmaleficence. The supervisor might suggest that by cosigning Bob's notes more people would have access to physical therapy services. If Laura accepts this argument, she must balance the benefit of increased access against the harm that might result from cosigning the notes. However, the supervisor would be stretching the boundaries of the concept to argue that beneficence could include fraudulent claims and exposing patients to possible risks from treatment by an unqualified provider. To do so would stretch the usual meaning of promoting good. To pose this solution to the problem would represent a utilitarian argument that cosigning the notes represents the greatest good for the greatest number (see Chapter 1).

Step 4: Prioritize values where conflicts exist   Can the conflicts between principles be identified? How should these duties, obligations, and virtues be prioritized? As suggested, this can be accomplished by using the principles of beneficence and nonmaleficence.

Step 5: Moral creativity and ingenuity   Are there solutions to the problem that embrace apparently competing duties? Is it possible to determine a course of action that allows apparently conflicting goals to be fulfilled? For example, can Laura design staffing options with her supervisor that allow her to supervise Bob as a technician? It may be that Laura, Bob, and a physical therapist assistant (PTA) could organize patient care so that all patients receive appropriate, safe, and legal care at a cost acceptable to the supervisor.

Step 6: Choose, implement, and reassess   If Laura chooses the option of attempting to cover all of the patients through creative staffing and teamwork, it will be important to plan the implementation and reassessment of her decision. It may be possible for the team to work out a plan for patient care that includes specific types of responsibility performed by each staff member, contingencies for her absence, and a set time to reassess how the plan is working.

LEGAL ANALYSIS

In general, state practice acts govern the provision of professional services. Their purpose is protection of the public through assurance of a minimum standard for licensees. They set forth who may obtain a license, what licensees are permitted to do with the license, and how the license can be lost. The major elements include a definition of the scope of practice; requirements for licensure, either by examination or through reciprocity; actions for which the board may impose discipline; and appointment of and duties of the licensing board.

The definition enumerates and delineates the scope of physical therapy practice. PTs should be aware of this definition and ensure that it is in accord with current therapy practice. For example, the APTA Board of Directors urges that the definition be broadly inclusive, not merely an enumeration of techniques (see the Appendix at the end of this chapter).[39] Definition language such as "including but not limited to" provides a means to incorporate new tests and techniques.

The Model Practice Act for Physical Therapy, produced by the Model Practice Act Task Force of the Federation of State Boards of Physical Therapy, recommends separating the definitions of physical therapy, PT, and the practice of physical therapy as follows[40]:

"Physical Therapy" means the care and services provided by or under the direction and supervision of a physical therapist licensed by this state. "Physical Therapist" means a person who meets all the requirements of this act, and is licensed in this state to practice physical therapy. The "Practice of Physical Therapy" means:

1. Examining, evaluating and testing individuals with mechanical, physiological and developmental impairments, functional limitations, and disability or other health and movement-related conditions in order to determine a diagnosis, prognosis, a plan of therapeutic intervention, and to assess the ongoing effects of intervention.
2. Alleviating impairments and functional limitations by designing, implementing, and modifying therapeutic interventions that include but are not limited to: therapeutic exercise, functional training in self care and in home, community or work reintegration, manual therapy including soft tissue and joint mobilization and manipulation, therapeutic massage, assistive and adaptive orthotic, prosthetic, protective and supportive devices and equipment, bronchopulmonary hygiene, debridement and wound care, physical agents or modalities, mechanical and electrotherapeutic modalities, and patient-related instruction.
3. Reducing the risk of injury, impairments, functional limitations and disability, including the promotion and maintenance of fitness, health and quality of life in all age populations.
4. Engaging in administration, consultation, education and research.

The definition language is critical in determining who may be permitted to practice physical therapy. The Arkansas Chiropractic Association instituted litigation to urge insurers not to pay for manipulation or mobilization techniques performed by physical therapists (personal communication, Bill Bandy, president of the Arkansas chapter of APTA, July 17, 1997). The Arkansas chapter of the APTA has since intervened in the litigation. Concurrently, the chapter sought changes in the definition of physical therapy within the state practice act. In 1997, the Arkansas state legislature adopted a definition of physical therapy that includes mobilization but excludes manipulation.[41]

Some states provide criminal or civil penalties for individuals who practice physical therapy without a physical therapy license. However, despite the existence of a statute expressly prohibiting chiropractors from representing themselves as physical therapists,[42] the Pennsylvania chapter of the APTA has been engaged in complex litigation surrounding the issue of chiropractors' right to advertise, provide, and bill for physical therapy services.[43] A prosecutor for the state board of physical therapy brought an action against a chiropractor for advertising that he performed "physical therapy" in his practice. (The Pennsylvania Physical Therapy Association later intervened on the side of the prosecution.) An administrative law judge concluded that the Chiropractic Practice Act, while preventing a chiropractor from representing him- or herself as a licensed physical therapist, "does not prohibit a chiropractor from practicing physical therapy."[43] The judge determined that the definition of "adjunctive procedures" under the Chiropractic Practice Act contained language identical to the definition of "physical therapy" under the Physical Therapy Act. The judge relied on a 1985 decision of the Superior Court of Pennsylvania,[44] which held that chiropractors may use (and bill for) modalities of treatment defined as physical therapy in treating misaligned vertebrae. The judge also looked to the language of the Physical Therapy Act prohibiting others from using the terms *physical therapy* or *physical therapist* "provided, however, That [sic] nothing in this section shall limit … a chiropractor's authority to practice chiropractic or to bill for such practice."[45]

Requirements for licensure can be supplemented by regulations promulgated by the licensure board. In general, therapists must successfully complete an examination or hold licensure in another state. States can also require that applicants demonstrate evidence of good moral character through such requirements as character references and disclosure of prior convictions. If a negative determination on a licensure application is based on such arguably subjective criteria, the licensee may be granted a hearing to contest an adverse determination.

Disciplinary provisions vary; some are rather broad, whereas others are specific. Courts have generally upheld state licensure board actions even in cases in which the language used to discipline a licensee has been rather vague, such as for "unprofessional conduct." For example, a PT's license was revoked in 1940 for creation of a public nuisance because of operation of a house of prostitution.[46] Some states also incorporate by reference the APTA *Guide for Professional Conduct*.

Several states have considered (and rejected) measures to do away with professional licensure for PTs. It is critical that PTs educate legislators regarding the purposes of licensure—that is, the protection of the public through ensuring adequately qualified health professionals.

Another critical issue addressed in the practice act is the scope of direct access. Some states permit evaluation and treatment without physician referral; others permit evaluation only. As reported by Mitchell and Lissovoy,[47]* 30 states permit PT evaluation and treatment without physician referral and 14 states permit evaluation. The type of practitioner who may refer a patient to a PT is also specified. Defining the parameters of direct access has been an issue for PTs for many years. In 1933, a PT was convicted of practicing medicine without a license.[48]

---

*The authors found that physical therapy delivered under direct access was of shorter duration and less costly than care delivered under physician referral.

The therapist was apparently assessing patients and subsequently telephoning a physician (not the patient's physician) for a referral.

The importance of the definition of physical therapy and the state's position with respect to direct access is illustrated in the following cases. In *Bolton v. CNS Ins. Co.*,[48] the Tennessee Supreme Court determined that a PT cannot testify regarding a patient's ultimate disability. In so doing, the court looked to the state practice act (which permits evaluation, but not treatment, without referral) and the accompanying legislative history, concluding that "physical therapy is a narrow health specialty limited in scope."[49] This case has been subsequently followed by courts in Tennessee and elsewhere to restrict the scope of PT expert testimony.[50] The Bolton case was cited in a case in Indiana,[51] in which it was argued that a PT is not competent to give an opinion on the permanence and extent of a patient's disability. The PT in this case was permitted to testify about her evaluation of the patient but could not testify about her treatment plan or goals that the patient's strength and coordination could be improved to the point that he could resume light farming duties.

In Laura's case, one must look to the state practice act and to any supporting rules and regulations issued by the licensing board to determine whether the proposed arrangement represents a violation of state law. Under the state law, Bob must surrender his temporary license. In that case, presumably he would function at the level of a technician, unless state law has another explicit category for such individuals (i.e., extension of student status during multiple examination attempts). Ongoing evaluation of patients would therefore be inappropriate, and the therapist cosigning the notes may be deemed to be contributing to the unlicensed practice of physical therapy, which may itself violate the practice act. It appears that some level of treatment under the supervision of the licensed therapist may be appropriate, again subject to the specifications contained within state law and regulations regarding direct supervision of nonlicensed personnel. Violation of these requirements may lead to criminal penalties and licensure sanctions, such as revocation or probation, depending on state law.

QUESTIONS AND NOTES FOR FURTHER REFLECTION

1. The issue of mandatory continuing education requirements is also addressed in the practice act or accompanying regulations. Twenty-one states have some form of continuing education mandate for PTs. Is mandatory continuing education a good idea for PTs?[52]

2. An alternative to a mandatory continuing education requirement is mandatory relicensure for health care professionals, in

which licensees must demonstrate evidence of current competency; is this preferable?

3. If Laura's supervisor told her that she would lose her job if she refused to cosign Bob's notes, would that change the ethical analysis?

4. Is the dilemma between cosigning the notes and refusing and being fired an ethical dilemma?

5. What are other possible solutions to Laura's situation?

6. What would you do if you knew of a clinic where they were practicing in this manner?

7. What is your state's position regarding direct access? Are any changes warranted?

Laura's case illustrates the difficulties faced by clinical facilities in managing heavy patient loads with limited staffing and financial resources. This case highlights issues posed by delegation of physical therapy services.

CASE 2.3

Linda Wilson is a PT technician in a rural general hospital; she is taking courses at the local community college and plans to become a PTA. Her supervisor, the physical therapy department director, oversees one PT, one PTA, and three PT technicians. The department provides inpatient and outpatient services and staffs a home health care agency operated by the hospital. One busy afternoon, the department director approaches Linda with a request. The PT is out sick, and the PTA is on vacation. The director asks Linda to visit a home health patient on her way home. The patient has not been evaluated by a PT, but Linda's boss tells her, "She's just a simple hip fracture; you know what to do." This is not the first time that the director has made such a request. What legal and ethical issues are raised by this situation?

Both Linda's situation and Laura's case deal with issues of professional roles and ethics. Both cases deal with the issue of proper supervision and delegation of duties by the PT, and both cases also involve working outside the legal restrictions on physical therapy practice. Finally, both cases involve the possible violation of the *Code of Ethics* and *Guide for Professional Conduct* with regard to appropriate supervision of support staff. The major difference between the cases is the professional or nonprofessional roles of the individuals involved and the specific context of the case. However, Linda's position as a nonlicensed technician serving in a nonprofessional capacity creates a power relationship that changes the context. Does Linda's boss have more responsibility than Linda because he is a professional? What are the obligations of professionals? What does it mean to be a professional?

ROLE OF PROFESSIONS IN MEDICINE

Medicine and law are two of the three historic professions: law, medicine, and theology. The meaning of the term *professional* is the subject of current debates, particularly with regard to their role in the field of medicine. The term *profession* comes from the Latin word *profiteor,* which means to profess a faith. As Purtilo and Haddad[54] noted, from this perspective "[a] profession is basically a calling that requires specialized knowledge and generally extensive academic preparation." The religious underpinnings of the words *profess* and *calling* suggest that being a professional involves a commitment to living out a certain kind of value system. Traditional discussions of the professions have focused on the characteristics that define a profession. The following qualities are also traditionally used to define a profession:

- Organized body of specialized knowledge*
- Code of ethics and standards of practice that members enforce through peer review
- Some degree of autonomy in making judgments†
- Accountability to society

Noting that there is no agreement about the definition of the word *profession,* Daniel Wueste[54] identified five general characteristics of professionals:

1. Centrality of abstract knowledge in performing their duties.
2. Social significance of the tasks. Professionals perform important social functions.

---

*At a conference discussion, one PT educator argued that doctoral education has been traditionally associated with recognition as a profession. Debate about the appropriate degree to award in the field of physical therapy implicitly is about how much education is necessary to acquire the specialized body of knowledge of physical therapy.

†Whether autonomy is a prerequisite for being a professional has been a source of debate in physical therapy. The opinion has been advanced by some that PTAs are paraprofessionals rather than professionals. Indeed, House of Delegates Policy 06-96-24-39 refers to PTs as "professionals" and PTAs as "paraprofessionals." At the same time, it can be argued that PTs themselves are not professionals because they do not have autonomy in their decisions as they act on physicians' orders in many cases. However, physical therapists have experienced increasing levels of autonomy as more and more states enact direct access legislation.

3. Claim that the professional is uniquely qualified.
4. Governed by role-specific norms rather than the norms of daily life.
5. Tendency to work within bureaucratic institutions.

Although the professions have historically been viewed in a positive light, some recent literature is critical of the professions. Whereas traditional notions of the professions emphasized ethical codes, journals, and educational requirements, this literature describes professions as interest groups protecting economic self-interest through specialized knowledge.[55] These critiques reinforce the social obligation of professions. Although all organizations have legitimate self-interests, it is particularly important for professions to fulfill their obligations to work for the common good.

Pellegrino and Thomasma[56] see in the current professional milieu a need to "reconcile two opposing orders—one based on the primacy of [medicine's] covenant with patients and the other based on the ethos of self-interest." The resolution to this dilemma, according to Pellegrino and Thomasma, resides in health care providers' ability to build a moral community.

> We wish to argue that medicine is at heart a moral community and always will be; that those who practice it are *de facto* members of a moral community, bound together by knowledge and ethical precepts; and that, as a result, [medical professionals] have collective, as well as individual, moral obligations to protect the welfare of sick persons in a world that increasingly treats medicine as a commodity, a political bauble, an investment opportunity, or a bureaucrat's power play.[55]

How do professions influence their members, the profession, institutions, and society in general? Although the mechanisms through which influence occurs are complex, professions basically achieve influence by shaping ideas, values, and regulatory policies. W. Richard Scott,[57] an organizational theorist, noted that professions accomplish this by defining reality for members.

The APTA develops standards, guidelines, positions, and policies. The APTA House of Delegates has the primary responsibility for leading the association through its actions, statements, and policy formulation. These statements assist members in formulating professional identity; they define the areas over which PTs have jurisdiction; and they delineate what PTs do and ought to be doing through guidelines and standards. In addition, the APTA works through political activity to position the profession within society as a whole. Because the APTA House of Delegates is made up of elected representatives, these positions represent a kind of consensus within the profession.

LEGAL ANALYSIS

Federal Law

Medicare has coverage guidelines for outpatient physical therapy services not provided in physicians' offices.[58] In addition to requiring specific standards, regulations mandate that the PT, as the practice owner, be present in the clinic whenever physical therapy services are rendered.[59] Because the regulations do not apply to physicians, questions of inappropriate delegation have arisen in this context. A 1994 study by the Office of the Inspector General of the U.S. Department of Health and Human Services found that many physicians are billing Medicare for physical therapy services provided by unlicensed personnel.[60] The APTA has been actively seeking to overturn these provisions.[61, 62] The Outpatient Physical Therapy Standards Act of 1997 was passed by Congress as part of the federal budget agreement.[60] The bill requires that services be restorative and reasonable (including frequency of services), that services relate to an identified care plan and goals, and that services require the skilled intervention of a physical therapist.

In the home health area, federal regulations mandate a PT site visit for patients treated by a PTA every 30 days.[62] However, some intermediaries require site visits as frequently as once per week (personal communication, Gail Grotsch, APTA Department of Government Affairs, February 20, 1997).

State Law

Some state practice acts explicitly address the issue of permissible delegation. For example, the Arizona physical therapy practice act provides that "no person shall work as a physical therapy aide, physical therapy attendant or physical therapy assistant except under the on-site supervision of a physical therapist."[63] Others do so through regulations by the state licensure board under authority granted in the practice act. Under regulations issued by the Tennessee licensure board, for example, all physical therapy evaluations must be performed by a licensed PT.* Furthermore, the state requires that therapy services provided by a technician be given under the direct (defined as "on-site") supervision of a PT or PTA.† Thus, in both Arizona and Tennessee, the

---

*Note that the APTA House of Delegates recommendation is that the supervising therapist be in the immediate area.

†For example, see Tennessee Rules and Regulations 1150-2-.10(2), which defines direct supervision in physical therapy.

director in Linda's case would be in violation of the state practice act for inappropriate delegation. Furthermore, he would be liable for any injury to the patient that arose from improper care of the patient by the technician. The model practice act developed by the Federation of State Boards of Physical Therapy suggests that a PT should not supervise more than three assistive personnel; the act leaves to states' discretion whether the term *assistive personnel* refers to PTAs or solely to unlicensed personnel.[41] The model act suggests that PT aides have continuous on-site supervision with the therapist immediately available to assist the aide.

The importance of clarifying permissible delegation through statute or regulations is illustrated by a recent situation in Vermont.[64] In May 1996, the counsel for Vermont's secretary of state initiated an inquiry into the physical therapy aide use. The secretary interpreted the state practice act to permit only a PT or PTA to be involved in any part of physical therapy. The Vermont chapter of the APTA succeeded in convincing the legislature to amend the practice act, clarifying that PTs may continue to use unlicensed physical therapy aides.

PTs can also be sanctioned under the relevant state practice act for aiding and abetting the unlicensed practice of physical therapy or medicine. Such violations may result in licensure restrictions. In 1948, a New York PT was suspended for 1 year for aiding the practice of physical therapy by unlicensed personnel.[65] More recently, a South Carolina PT was charged by the state board of physical therapy examiners with unprofessional conduct for allowing unregistered persons to perform physical therapy and for inadequate documentation.[66] The therapist had instructed his nonlicensed employees to perform massage, hotpack application, ultrasound, gait training, traction, whirlpool, and electrical stimulation although he was not present for the treatments. The employees also documented treatment notes for the procedures.

Where state law does not address appropriate delegation parameters, courts look to the industry standard to determine if the actions of the therapist are reasonable. In Linda's case, the APTA *Standards of Practice for Physical Therapy* and *Guide for Professional Conduct*, as well as published opinions of the APTA Board of Directors, all indicate that the director acted outside the permissible standard of physical therapy delegation.

QUESTIONS AND NOTES FOR FURTHER REFLECTION

1. Situations may be envisioned that are not as clear cut as Linda's case. For example, does on-site supervision include all areas of a campus of a large medical center, even though they may be located several blocks apart?

2. Should specific delegation parameters, such as supervision ratios, be established? Should they vary by practice setting? Should they be recommendations or carry the force of law? What exceptions might apply, if any?

3. In a 1993 study, 67% of therapists surveyed indicated that aide use had presented them with ethical dilemmas at some time.[66]

4. What differences exist between professionals and nonprofessionals in providing physical therapy?

5. In what ways is the profession of physical therapy a moral community?

CASE FOR FURTHER REFLECTION

Tom Hudson is the PT in an extended care facility. From 8 AM until 2 PM Tom sees patients in the facility, and in the afternoons he sees a small number of patients in the home health service owned by the facility. Tom supervises a PTA and PT technician at the facility. A large percentage of Tom's patient load involves whirlpool treatments and wound debridement. One morning, Tom arrives at work to discover that the PTA, who normally supervises the PT technician in performing whirlpool treatments, has undergone emergency surgery during the night. She will be out of work for 10 weeks. The physical therapy department has the following work to accomplish: six new evaluations, seven whirlpool treatments, 10 exercise sessions, and 12 gait-training sessions. Tom also has three home health patients to see. It occurs to him that one solution is for the PT technician to see the whirlpool patients and the gait-training patients while Tom is seeing home health patients. What issues are raised by this delegation of responsibility?

REFERENCES

1. Black's Law Dictionary (4th ed). St. Paul, MN: West, 1979.
2. *McCay v. Mitchell*, 463 S.W.2d 710, 62 Tenn. App. 424 (1970).
3. Tenn. Code Ann. 63-6-218.
4. *Wade v. John D. Archbold Memorial Hospital*, 252 Ga. 118, 311 S.E.2d 836 (1984).
5. Gresham GE, Duncan PW, Stason WB, et al. Post-Stroke Rehabilitation. Clinical Practice Guideline, no. 16. Public Health Service, Agency for Health Care Policy and Research Publication 95-0662. Rockville, MD: U.S. Dept. of Health and Human Services, 1995.
6. *Ybarra v. Spangard*, 25 Cal.2d 486, 154 P.2d 687 (1944).

7. *St. Paul Fire and Marine Insurance Company v. Prothro*, 266 Ark. 1020, 590 S.W.2d 35 (1979).
8. *Gilles v. Rehabilitation Institute of Oregon*, 498 P.2d 777 (Or. 1972).
9. *Hendley v. Springhill Memorial Hospital and West Mobile Therapy Assoc.*, 575 So.2d 547 (Ala. 1990).
10. *Darling v. Charleston Community Memorial Hospital*, 33 Ill.2d 326, 211 N.E.2d 253 (1965), cert. denied 383 U.S. 946 (1966).
11. *Zucker v. Axelrod*, 527 N.Y.S.2d 937, 139 A.D.2d 966 (A.D.4 Dept. 1988).
12. Risk Management Pearls for Physical Therapists. A Project of the Committee on Risk Management Services and Member Benefits of APTA in Cooperation with the American Society for Healthcare Risk Management. Alexandria, VA: American Physical Therapy Association, 1996;3.
13. American Heritage College Dictionary (3rd ed). Boston: Houghton-Mifflin, 1993;127.
14. Thiroux JP. Ethics: Theory and Practice (5th ed). Englewood Cliffs, NJ: Prentice-Hall, 1995;182.
15. Arras JD, Steinbock B. Ethical Issues in Modern Medicine (4th ed). Mountain View, CA: Mayfield, 1995;21.
16. Miller BL. Autonomy and the Refusal of Lifesaving Treatment. Hastings Center Report 1981;11:22–28.
17. Beauchamp TL, Childress JF. Principles of Biomedical Ethics (4th ed). New York: Oxford University Press, 1994;123.
18. MacIntyre A. After Virtue (2nd ed). Notre Dame, IN: Notre Dame Press, 1984;60, 194.
19. Jennings B. Healing the self: the moral meaning of relationships in rehabilitation. Am J Phys Med Rehabil 1993;72:401–404.
20. AMA Center for Health Policy Research. Trends in U.S. Health Care 1992. Chicago: American Medical Association, 1992;130.
21. Weiler P, Hiatt H, Newhouse J, et al. A Measure of Malpractice. Cambridge, MA: Harvard University Press, 1993;55.
22. Study claims malpractice actions drop. PT Bull June 15, 1994;4.
23. Weiler P. Medical Malpractice on Trial. Cambridge, MA: Harvard University Press, 1991;4.
24. Fellechner B, Findley T. Malpractice in physical medicine and rehabilitation. A review and analysis of existing data. Am J Phys Med Rehabil 1991;70:124.
25. Scott R. Health Care Malpractice. Thorofare, NJ: Slack, 1990;3.
26. Scott R. Malpractice update. PT Mag 1996;4:69.
27. Reichley M. What every PT should know about liability insurance. Advance Phys Therapists, October 24, 1994;6.
28. Horsh D. Medico-Legal Aspects of Physical Therapy. In R Hickok (ed), Physical Therapy Administration and Management. Baltimore: Williams & Wilkins, 1974.
29. Pozgar G. Legal Aspects of Health Care Administration (5th ed). Gaithersburg, MD: Aspen, 1993.
30. Health Lawyers News 1997;1:9.
31. Health Care Quality Improvement Act of 1986. 42 U.S.C.A. §11101 et seq.
32. Reporting Medical Malpractice Payments. 45 C.F.R. §60.7(a).
33. Reporting Medical Malpractice Payments. 45 C.F.R. §60.7(d).

34. Information Which Hospitals Must Request from the National Practitioner Data Bank. 45 C.F.R. §60.10.
35. Kadzielski M. The National Practitioner Data Bank: big brother or paper tiger? Healthspan 1992;9:8.
36. Office of the Inspector General, U.S. Department of Health and Human Services. National Health Lawyers News Report [draft] 1995;23:5.
37. Massachusetts Board of Registration in Medicine. National Health Lawyer's News Report 1997;24:6.
38. An Act to Redefine the Terms Physical Therapist, Physical Therapy Practice and Physical Therapy Aide; and for Other Purposes. Act 744 (1977), adding Ark. code 17.93-313.
39. Board of Directors, American Physical Therapy Association. Model Definition of "Physical Therapy." Alexandria, VA: American Physical Therapy Association, 1995.
40. The Federation of State Boards of Physical Therapy. The Model Practice Act for Physical Therapy. Alexandria, VA: The Federation of State Boards of Physical Therapy, 1997.
41. An Act to Redefine the Terms Physical Therapist, Physical Therapy Practice and Physical Therapy Aide; and for Other Purposes. Act 744 (1977), amending Ark. code 17-93-102.
42. 63 Penn. Stat. §625.526(b).
43. *Pennsylvania Bureau of Professional Affairs v. Boch,* Nos. 0085-65-95, 0460-65-95, 0456-65-95, 00457-65-95 (Pa. Bd. of Physical Therapy, Jan. 2, 1997).
44. *Allstate Insurance Co. v. Williams,* 500 A.2d 1151 (Pa. Super. 1985).
45. 63 Penn. Stat. §1304 (b.1).
46. *Swift v. Graves,* 19 N.Y.S.2d 686 (Sup. Ct. 1940).
47. Mitchell J, deLissovoy G. A comparison of resource use and cost in direct access versus physician referral episodes of physical therapy. Phys Ther 1997;77:10.
48. *People v. Mari,* 260 N.Y. 389, 183 N.E. 858 (1933).
49. *Bolton v. CNS Ins. Co.,* 821 S.W.2d 932 (Tenn. 1991).
50. *Bailey v. Colonial Freight Systems, Inc.,* 836 S.W.2d 554 (Tenn. 1992).
51. *Stutzman v. CRST, Inc.* 997 F.2d 291 (7th Cir. 1993).
52. Hruska R, Harden B. Should continuing education be a requirement for relicensure? PT Mag 1994;2:72.
53. Purtilo R, Haddad A. Health Professional and Patient Interaction (5th ed). Philadelphia: Saunders, 1996;11, 100.
54. Wueste DE (ed). Professional Ethics and Social Responsibility. Lanham, MD: Rowman & Littlefield, 1994;11.
55. Macdonald KM. The Sociology of the Professions. London: Sage Publications, 1995;30.
56. Pellegrino ED, Thomasma DC. The Virtues in Medical Practice. New York: Oxford University Press, 1993;31, 32.
57. Scott WR. Institutions and Organizations. Thousand Oaks, CA: Sage Publications, 1995;95.
58. Conditions for Coverage: Outpatient Physical Therapy Services Furnished by Physical Therapists in Independent Practice, 42 C.F.R. 486.150–163.
59. Conditions for Coverage: Supervision, 42 C.F.R. 486.151.
60. Outpatient Physical Therapy Standards Act of 1997 could save Medicare millions annually. PT Bull, May 16, 1997;11.

61. Congress acts on private practice supervision concerns. PT Bull, October 25, 1996;13.
62. Conditions of Participation: Physical Therapy Services, 42 C.F.R. 485.713(a)(2)(ii).
63. Ariz. Rev. Stat. Ann. Section 32-2041 (D).
64. Shiratori S. Vermont PTs salvage physical therapist aide utilization; regulation of other personnel being discussed. PT Bull 1997;12:8.
65. *O'Neill v. Board of Regents of Univ of State of N.Y.*, 298 N.Y. 777, 83 N.E.2d 469 (1948).
66. *Huba v. S.C. State Board of Physical Therapy Examiners*, 446 S.E.2d 433 (S.C. 1994).
67. Laden Bashi H, Domholdt E. Use of support personnel for physical therapy treatment. Phys Ther 1993;73:421.

Appendix

Model Definition of Physical Therapy for State Practice Acts*

Physical therapy, which is the care and services provided by or under the direction and supervision of a physical therapist, includes:

1. examining (history, system review and tests and measure) individuals with impairment, functional limitation, and disability or other health-related conditions in order to determine a diagnosis, prognosis, and intervention; tests and measures include, but are not limited to, the following:

   aerobic capacity or endurance
   anthropometric characteristics
   arousal, mentation, and cognition
   assistive and adaptive devices
   community and work (job/school/play) integration/reintegration
   cranial nerve integrity
   environmental, home and work (job/school/play) barriers
   ergonomics and body mechanics
   gait, locomotion, and balance
   integumentary integrity
   joint integrity and mobility
   motor function
   muscle performance
   neuromotor development and sensory integration
   orthotic, protective and supportive devices
   pain

*Reprinted from Model Definition of Physical Therapy for State Practice Acts BOD 02-97-03-06 (Program 19) [Amended BOD 03-95-24-64; BOD 06-94-03-04; BOD 03-93-18-46]. Board of Directors Professional and Societal Policies, Positions, and Guidelines. Alexandria, VA: American Physical Therapy Association, 1997.

posture
prosthetic requirements
range of motion
reflex integrity
self-care and home-management
sensory integrity
ventilation, respiration, and circulation

2. alleviating impairment and functional limitation by designing, implementing, and modifying therapeutic interventions that include, but are not limited to:

coordination, communication, and documentation
patient-related instruction
therapeutic exercise (including aerobic conditioning)
functional training in self-care and home-management (including activities of daily living and instrumental activities of daily living)
functional training in community and work (job/school/play) integration/reintegration activities (including instrumental activities of daily living, work hardening, and work conditioning)
manual therapy techniques (including mobilization and manipulation)
prescription, application, and, as appropriate fabrication of assistive, adaptive, orthotic, protective, supportive, and prosthetic devices and equipment
airway clearance techniques
wound management
electrotherapeutic modalities
physical agents and mechanical modalities

3. preventing injury, impairment, functional limitation, and disability, including the promotion and maintenance of fitness, health, and quality of life in all age populations
4. engaging in consultation, education and research

3

Business Issues

Medical practice and medical ethics developed in the United States within assumed contextual parameters that are now being challenged. Some of these contextual parameters are fee-for-service reimbursement; the inviolability of the patient-physician relationship; and not-for-profit, community-based hospitals. Although Medicare and the increasing availability of insurance through employers means that practicing medicine can be lucrative, medicine continues to be viewed as a service profession rather than a business. With medical costs soaring and the national debt rising, avenues for cost containment are being explored.

One suggested approach to cost containment is to adopt a business model for health care delivery. Viewing medical practice and physical therapy practice from a business perspective presents a major challenge to traditional medical, ethical, and legal perspectives. By suggesting a fundamental shift in the context within which medical care is provided, the business perspective represents a break with previous models of medicine. This paradigm shift offers both challenges and opportunities for physical therapy. (Of course, there has always been tension between medicine as a service profession and medicine as a business. It can be argued that current trends merely represent an exaggeration of preexisting tendencies in the industry.) This chapter explores the ongoing tensions and challenges that viewing medicine primarily as a business presents.

The chapter begins with a case that examines the legal and ethical issues raised by advertising. The mechanisms for pursuing a claim of violation of the American Physical Therapy Association's (APTA) *Code of Ethics* are described in this context. The problems associated with personal or financial incentives for over- or underutilization of health care services are then discussed. These problems reflect the difficulty that the shift to a business perspective creates for the relationship between health care provider and patient. This idea is explored from the perspective of changes in the traditional concept of the relationship between physician and patient. Overall, financial incentives for levels of care and the changing relationship between patient and provider inherent in managed care suggest the need for increased accountability in the health care system. Models of accountability in the managed care age are addressed. The chapter concludes with a discussion of some of the legal issues presented by managed care.

CASE 3.1

Linda Waller owns a private practice that focuses on hand therapy. She experienced a decline in her patient base when the local hospital hired a certified hand therapist. Although Linda has had significant training and experience treating hand patients, she has never taken the time to become certified. Linda decided to advertise her practice to try to increase public awareness of her services and to recapture the referrals of the orthopedic surgeons in the area. She placed the following advertisement:

WALLER THERAPY CLINIC
Hand therapy specialist. 15 years
of providing the best hand therapy in the region.

The advertisement included before and after photos of a patient with a particularly complex crush-injury with whom Linda achieved an unusually good result. In addition to the advertisement, Linda wrote a column describing the services offered by her clinic and paid the community newspaper to print the column; it was not identified as paid advertising.

What legal and ethical issues are raised by the placement of this advertisement? Suppose that the certified hand therapist at the hospital, Frieda Findlay, reads Linda's advertisement. She is incensed that Linda would represent herself as a hand therapist, especially when Frieda thinks about how long she studied to become a certified hand therapist. Frieda believes that Linda has engaged in unethical behavior and resolves to file a complaint with the ethics committee of the state chapter of the APTA. How should she go about this?

ADVERTISING ISSUES

Traditionally, medical and legal professionals have not advertised their services. Medical advertisements were considered inherently misleading as the consumer lacked knowledge of medicine and necessarily relied on the expertise of the physician to make an appropriate referral. Advertising was thus viewed as unprofessional and, in fact, unethical. Until the 1970s, many professional associations' codes of ethics contained a provision expressly prohibiting advertising by their members. In 1979, however, the Federal Trade Commission (FTC) brought suit against the American Medical Association (AMA), arguing that the AMA's ethical principles interfered with the physician's right to advertise and were thus a restraint of trade.[1] It is now well settled law that professional societies cannot prohibit truthful advertising because it is protected under antitrust laws as a means to ensure free trade. The rationale is to preserve and promote free and open competition by enabling professionals to disseminate information about their services to patients to help them make better informed judgments and choices.

Prohibition of advertising is also a Constitutional issue. Commercial speech is protected under the First Amendment, which guarantees the right to free speech. In *Virginia State Board of Pharmacy v. Virginia Citizens Consumer Council, Inc.*, the Supreme Court rejected Virginia's ban on price advertising for prescription drugs, which the state argued was necessary to maintain the professionalism of licensed pharmacists.[2] The Court sought to protect a free flow of information to consumers, noting, however, that this protection might be subject to certain limitations. For example, in a case involving an attorney's direct solicitation of accident victims, the Court found that the state had a legitimate and compelling interest in protecting the public from "those aspects of solicitation that involve fraud, undue influence, intimidation, overreaching, and other forms of 'vexatious conduct.'"[3]

The Federal Trade Commission Act[4] prohibits "unfair methods of competition in commerce" and "unfair or deceptive acts or practices in commerce," including misleading advertising. In addition to making only truthful representations, advertisers must disclose material facts. A material fact is one likely to affect the judgment of the average consumer at whom the advertisement is directed. Comparative references to competitors are permissible if they are truthful, but they must be clear and avoid deception.[5] With respect to patient endorsements, the experience of the individual should be representative of the experience of similar patients generally (and should not reflect a highly unusual best result). If an advertisement is found to be deceptive, the FTC can issue a cease-and-desist order, prohibiting further dissemination of the ad, and may require corrective advertising. If cease-and-desist orders are violated, the act provides for civil penalties.[6]

Under the Lanham Act, an individual may bring suit against a competitor for false advertising.[7] The typical remedy is to restrain the advertiser from further dissemination of the ad. In addition, competitors can file a complaint with the National Advertising Division of the Council of Better Business Bureaus (NAD).[8] Competitors can also bring suit for business disparagement or trade libel.[9, 10]

Many state practice acts also contain restrictions on false and misleading communications. For example, Hawaii's physical therapy practice act provides for disciplinary action for "making an untruthful and improbable statement in advertising one's practice of business" and "false, fraudulent, or deceptive advertising."[11] Violation of these provisions may subject a physical therapist (PT) to a range of licensure actions, such as probation or censure, depending on state law.

ANTITRUST LAWS

Advertising

Undue restrictions on advertising by professional societies are an example of the type of restraint of trade prohibited by antitrust laws. The primary purpose of antitrust laws, both federal and state, is to promote competition and free trade. Federal statutes, notably the Sherman Act, the Clayton Act, and the Federal Trade Commission Act, are enforced by the antitrust division of the U.S. Justice Department and the FTC. The Sherman Act prohibits restraint of trade and monopolization.[12] The Clayton Act prohibitions include price discrimination, exclusive dealing and tying, and monopolization.[13] The Federal Trade Commission Act provides that "unfair methods of competition in or affecting commerce, and unfair or deceptive acts or practices in or affecting commerce, are hereby declared unlawful."[14] Sanctions for violation of these provisions include fines (that can be quite substantial) and injunctions (restraining orders) prohibiting such conduct. Claims for damages can also be brought by individuals who are harmed by anticompetitive actions. In addition, many states have enacted antitrust laws. Antitrust enforcement in health care has been an area of focus for the FTC, which has released several policy statements regarding antitrust oversight in the health care industry. The next section discusses some common areas of antitrust enforcement in health care.

Health Care Applications

Health facility mergers are considered potential monopolies if the merger would result in control of a significant portion of market share. For example, the FTC brought suit against the Hospital Corporation of America (HCA), challenging the purchase of two hospital corporations in the Chattanooga, Tennessee, area.[15] The purchase would have given HCA control of 5 of 11 area hospitals. The FTC and the reviewing appellate court found that control of this proportion of the market was likely to foster collusive practices harmful to consumers. The theory is that such acquisitions may enable the acquiring company "to cooperate (or cooperate better) with other leading competitors on reducing or limiting output, thereby pushing up the market price."[15]

Other antitrust issues that arise in the health care area include restraint of trade and group boycotts (raised occasionally in hospital staff privileges disputes or with exclusive contracts), price fixing, and division of markets. Routine exclusion of a class of nonphysician providers from participation in a managed care organization (MCO) may constitute an antitrust violation if it can be shown to constitute an anticompetitive boycott.[16] The group boycott theory is illustrated in the case of *Wilk v. American Medical Association*, in which the FTC charged the AMA with a group boycott against chiropractors.[17]

A major area of potential litigation currently involves antitrust implications of networks. Networks are typically groups of physicians or, in some cases, multiple providers that aggregate to enjoy economies of scale and to market their services to MCOs or directly to employers. In general, a network must show integration to pass antitrust scrutiny— that is, a collection of providers must come together for a purpose other than "to show a united front" or to boycott managed care entities seeking to enter a local market. As early as 1942, the AMA and a local medical society were found guilty of violating the restraint of trade prohibitions of the Sherman Act. The groups orchestrated a boycott of a nonprofit corporation organized by government employees to provide medical care and hospitalization on a risk-sharing prepayment basis (Group Health).[18] The Supreme Court found that the defendants had coerced physicians into declining employment under Group Health, restrained AMA members from consulting with Group Health physicians, and restrained area hospitals from granting staff privileges to Group Health physicians.

In another case, the New York State Chiropractic Association agreed not to conspire in dealing with third-party payers; the complaint charged that the association conspired with its members to increase the level of reimbursement paid for chiropractic services by collectively threatening not to participate in a program of a third-party payer.[19]

The FTC has reviewed and given its approval to a number of physician networks. In August 1996, the U.S. Department of Justice and the FTC issued statements addressing physician and multiprovider networks.* The agencies indicated that they would not challenge exclusive physician networks whose physician participants share substantial financial risk and constitute 20% or fewer of physicians in each specialty who practice within the relevant geographic market (the threshold is 30% for nonexclusive networks). Presumably, such analysis will be applied similarly to physical therapy networks.

---

*Statement of the Antitrust Enforcement Policy in Health Care.

Application to Case 3.1

Although Linda clearly has a legal right to advertise, the advertisements as placed could be considered unfair or deceptive. The advertisement suggests that Linda is recognized by her peers as a specialist in hand therapy, although she has not, in fact, received certification. Furthermore, the testimonial photographs she has selected are not representative of typical results and, thus, may be deceptive. In addition, the column does not indicate that Linda paid for its placement, suggesting that the newspaper chose to profile her clinic and that the newspaper provided an objective assessment of services rather than the biased view offered by Linda.

Linda's competitor can choose to submit complaints to the FTC, the state's attorney general, the NAD, and the state licensing board. She can file a suit against Linda under the Lanham Act. If the column in the newspaper explicitly disparages the competitor, she might also sue Linda for trade disparagement or libel.* Linda may thus be subject to a restraining order that prohibits her from running the advertisement. She might also be subject to fines and to licensure sanctions.

PROCEDURES FOR CLAIMS OF UNETHICAL CONDUCT

Ways in which professional organizations shape the beliefs and actions of their members were discussed in Chapter 2. Professional organizations shape members' views by issuing statements and establishing guidelines for their members. The APTA publishes five documents that directly guide members in ethical matters (the association has established numerous policies related to ethical issues, but these documents represent the explicit position of the association on ethical matters). In deciding how she should proceed, therefore, Frieda might refer to the following resources.

---

*Although the case does not explicitly raise the issue, some competitor cases have resulted in libel and defamation lawsuits. See, for example, *The Georgia Society of Plastic Surgeons et al. v. Anderson et al.*, 363 S.E.2d 140, 257 Ga. 710 (1987). In this case, otolaryngologists and cosmetic surgeons brought suit against several physicians for libel and disparagement of services in a case arising from an article published in the state medical association journal. The article, by a plastic surgeon, was titled "Things Are Never What They Seem, Skim Milk Masquerades as Cream." In reference to the competitors' formation of a new medical society, the article stated, "If one's qualifications are shaky, the best conceivable smokescreen is to create a new organization with a high-sounding name, join it, issue yourself a certificate for display in your waiting room, and circulate the good news to all the medical societies in the country via a mass mailing." The plaintiffs in this case were awarded $500,000 in actual damages and $1,000,000 in punitive damages.

Code of Ethics

The *Code of Ethics* is the set of ethical principles that the APTA has decided should guide all PTs in their conduct. The APTA House of Delegates is the only body that may make changes to the *Code of Ethics*. The term *code of ethics* is reserved for exclusive use as the title of one document approved by the association's House of Delegates in accordance with the association's bylaws.[20]

Standards of Ethical Conduct

The *Standards of Ethical Conduct for the Physical Therapist Assistant* sets the guidelines for ethical conduct for physical therapist assistants (PTAs). Association definitions delineate that the standards are "an approved, binding statement used to judge quality of action or activity. The use of 'ethical standard' refers to right and wrong conduct." Table 3.1 outlines similarities and differences between the *Code* for PTs and the *Standards* for PTAs.

Guide for Professional Conduct

The *Guide for Professional Conduct of the American Physical Therapy Association* describes its purpose as "to serve physical therapists who are members of the American Physical Therapy Association (Association) in interpreting the *Code of Ethics* (Code) and matters of professional conduct."[21] The House of Delegates' policies define the term *guide* as "reserved for exclusive use in the titles of two documents issued by the Association's Judicial Committee in accordance with the Association's bylaws, i.e., the Guide for Professional Conduct and the Guide for Conduct of the Affiliate Member."[21]

It is helpful to remember the distinctions among the various association documents, because there are distinctions among levels of expected compliance. In addition to the *Code*, the *Guide*, and the *Standards*, the association publishes policies, positions, guidelines, and procedures. The House of Delegates Policies define them as follows[20]:

- Policy: A decision which obligates actions or subsequent decisions on similar matters.
- Position: An approved opinion or judgment which APTA members are expected to support.
- Guidelines: Approved, non-binding statements of advice.
- Procedure: Steps required to achieve a result.

Note that policies, positions, guidelines, procedures, guides, and standards call for different levels and types of obligations. For example, members are expected to verbalize support of and act in agreement with

Table 3.1
Similarities and differences between American Physical Therapy Association's *Code of Ethics for Physical Therapists* and *Standards of Ethical Conduct for the Physical Therapist Assistant*

Code of Ethics		Standards of Ethical Conduct for the Physical Therapist Assistant
Preamble "This *Code of Ethics* sets forth ethical principles for the physical therapy profession. Members of this profession are responsible for maintaining and promoting ethical practice. This *Code of Ethics* … shall be binding on PTs who are members of the Association."		**Preamble** "PTAs are responsible for maintaining and promoting high standards of conduct. These *Standards of Ethical Conduct for the PTA* shall be binding on PTAs who are affiliate members of the Association."
—	U →	**Standard 1** PTAs provide services under the supervision of a physical therapist.
Principle 1 PTs respect the rights and dignity of all individuals.	I	**Standard 2** PTAs respect the rights and dignity of all individuals.
Principle 4 PTs maintain and promote high standards for physical therapy practice, education, and research.	S	**Standard 3** PTAs maintain and promote high standards in the provision of services, giving the welfare of patients their highest regard.
Principle 2 PTs comply with the laws and regulations governing the practice of physical therapy.	S	**Standard 4** PTAs provide services within the limits of the law.
Principle 3 PTs accept responsibility for the exercise of sound judgment.	S	**Standard 5** PTAs make those judgments that are commensurate with their qualifications as PTAs.
Principle 7 PTs accept the responsibility to protect the public and the profession from unethical, incompetent, or illegal acts.	I	**Standard 6** PTAs accept the responsibility to protect the public and the profession from unethical, incompetent, or illegal acts.
Principle 5 PTs seek remuneration for their services that is deserved and reasonable.	U ←	—

Code of Ethics	Standards of Ethical Conduct for the Physical Therapist Assistant	
Principle 6	U	—
PTs provide accurate information to the consumer about the profession and about those services they provide.	←	
Principle 8		
PTs participate in efforts to address the health needs of the public.	U ←	—

U = unique to the *Code of Ethics* or to the *Standards of Ethical Conduct* (indicated by arrows); S = similar content and wording; I = identical content and wording; PTs = physical therapists; PTAs = physical therapist assistants.

policy statements of the APTA. However, guidelines do not obligate members to particular actions; they simply offer advice to members.

Professional obligations placed on members should be differentiated from obligations imposed by laws, regulatory standards, organizational guidelines, and the standards of third-party payers. Although the lines between these obligations are frequently blurred, it is important to distinguish the source and level of obligations. For example, PTs may be aware in daily practice that they are obligated to document patients' progress, including writing a discharge summary for each patient. It is important to know whether these obligations are to legal, private, organizational, or professional entities. For example, the organization for which I work may propose a shift to computer-based documentation. In that case, I must sort through obligations to determine the ramifications for physical therapy practice.

The *Guide* elaborates on each principle of the *Code*. Whereas the *Code* is a short document of broad ethical principles, the *Guide* describes specific behaviors that are consistent or inconsistent with the broader ethical principles. Remembering Beauchamp and Childress's distinction between principles and rules,[22] the *Code* provides principles of conduct whereas the *Guide* provides rules of conduct. Rules are more specific than principles. The *Guide* also delineates virtues and behaviors that are explicitly prohibited, encouraged, or allowed. For example, the first principle of the *Code* enjoins members to "respect the rights and dignity of all individuals."[21] In elaborating this principle of the *Code*, the *Guide* addresses attitudes of physical therapists, confidential information, patient relations, and informed consent. In describing the PT's obligation to respect the rights and dignity of his or her patients, some behaviors are prohibited, some are encouraged or required, and others are allowed.[22]

These distinctions between prohibition, requirement, and permission can be important in deciding whether a member has engaged in unethical behavior. When the *Guide* does not explicitly delineate that actions are required, allowed, or prohibited, decisions must be made based on the interpretation of the *Code* and the specific context in which the behavior occurred.

Although the *Guide* and *Standards* provide explicit attention to ethical behavior of members, members also have an implicit obligation to provide appropriate physical therapy intervention for patients. The APTA *Standards of Practice for Physical Therapy and the Clinical Accompanying Criteria*[23] provides a basis to judge whether physical therapy care is appropriate.

Guide for Conduct of the Affiliate Member

The *Guide* is intended to assist affiliate members in interpreting the *Standards*, similar to the manner in which the *Guide for Professional Conduct* interprets the *Code* for physical therapists. The APTA Judicial Committee, which is appointed by the board of the directors of the APTA, has responsibility for keeping the documents current with changes in the health care delivery system.

Procedural Document

The *Procedural Document on Disciplinary Action of the American Physical Therapy Association* lays out a "procedure to process claims that a member of the Association has violated" either the *Code* or *Standards*.[24] It outlines the steps to take in processing claims, and it delineates the rights and responsibilities of all participants in the process. The Judicial Committee has the responsibility for revising the procedural document.

Other Documents

In addition to these official documents of the APTA, the Judicial Committee provides other resources for members who serve in the disciplinary process, such as the *Compendium of Interpretations and Opinions*[25] and the *Investigation Guidelines for Chapter Ethics Committees of the American Physical Therapy Association*.[26] The general counsel of the APTA also provides sample letters for the various steps of the disciplinary process to the chairs of chapter ethics committees.

THE JUDICIAL PROCESS

The complete process for investigating an alleged ethical violation by a member of the APTA entails six major steps, as outlined in the *Procedural Document* and in Figure 3.1:

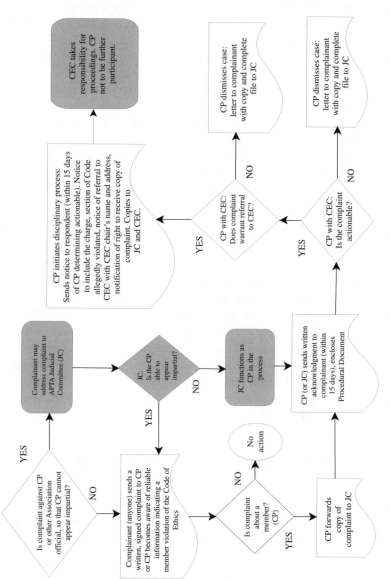

Figure 3.1 Steps in the disciplinary process. (APTA = American Physical Therapy Association; CP = chapter president; CEC = chapter ethics committee.)

1. Initiation of procedure by chapter president
2. Chapter ethics committee (CEC) conducts proceedings
3. CEC action
   a. Dismiss the charge against the respondent
   b. Recommend that the Judicial Committee take one of the following four actions: (1) reprimand, (2) probation, (3) suspension, (4) expulsion
4. Judicial Committee reviews CEC decision, including hearing if requested by respondent and decides to
   a. Impose the recommended CEC disciplinary action, specifying effective date
   b. Impose less severe penalties than CEC recommendation
   c. Dismiss the charges against the respondent
   d. Remand to the CEC with appropriate directives
5. Appeal to Board of Directors of the APTA
6. Postdecisional matters (monitoring and reviewing of suspension, publication of suspension, and expulsion decisions)

It is important to note that the disciplinary process can be used only with members of the association. The APTA is a voluntary association. Accordingly, the sanctions that it imposes relate to the rights and privileges of membership: probation, suspension, and expulsion from membership in the association. It is not uncommon for members to drop their membership before a final decision by the Judicial Committee.

The *Procedural Document* outlines specific steps to ensure that the rights of the individuals involved are protected and that timely and appropriate communication and documentation are maintained. Essentially, the process outlined in the *Procedural Document* ensures that due process is accorded to all participants. Figure 3.2 illustrates the process of filing a complaint.

CASE 3.1: FRIEDA FINDLAY'S COMPLAINT

Frieda Findlay believes that Linda Waller has engaged in unethical behavior through presenting herself as a specialist in hand therapy when she has no credentials commensurate with that claim. In deciding what she should do, Frieda can make use of the *Guide* and the *Procedural Document*. (She may also use other association policies, standards, or documents.) Many chapters publish these documents in the member directory, or they can be obtained through the APTA. In this case, Frieda calls the chapter president directly. Frieda need not be a member to file a complaint against a member of the association. Anyone may file a complaint. The chapter president informs Frieda that in

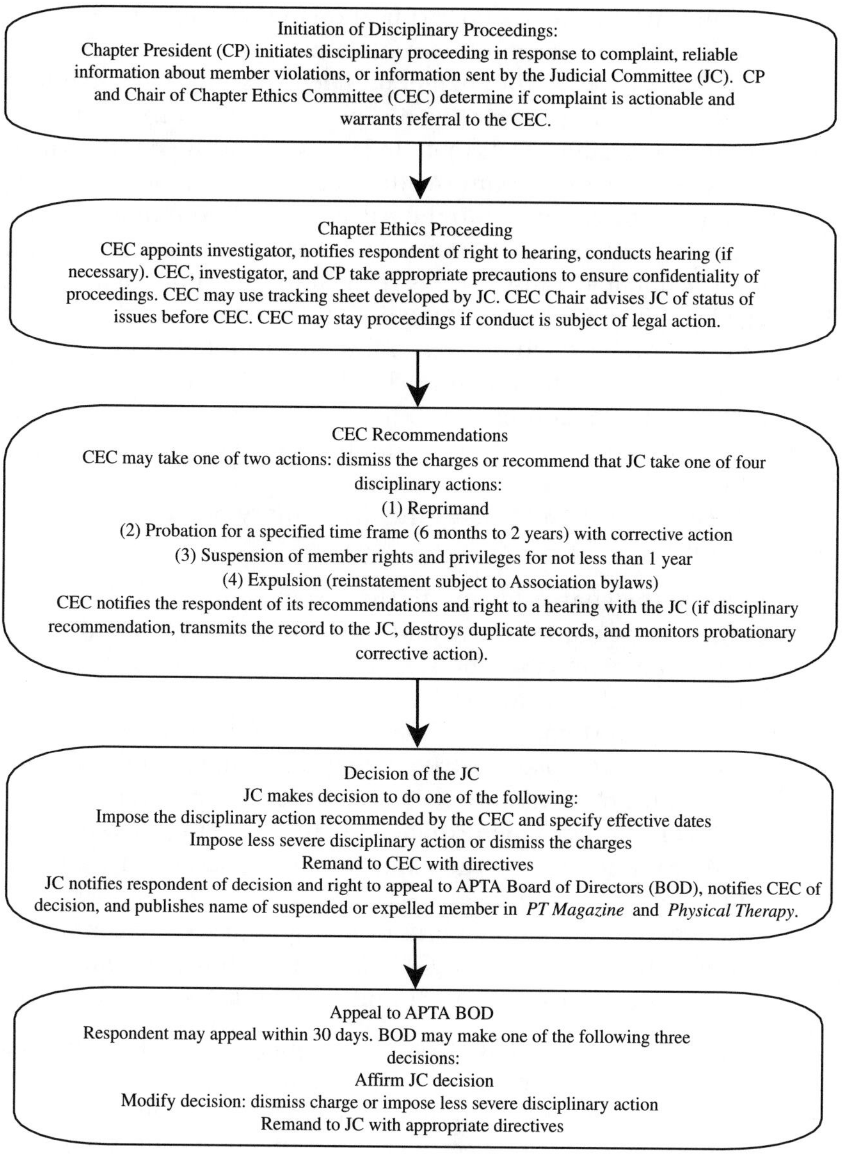

Initiation of Disciplinary Proceedings:
Chapter President (CP) initiates disciplinary proceeding in response to complaint, reliable information about member violations, or information sent by the Judicial Committee (JC). CP and Chair of Chapter Ethics Committee (CEC) determine if complaint is actionable and warrants referral to the CEC.

Chapter Ethics Proceeding
CEC appoints investigator, notifies respondent of right to hearing, conducts hearing (if necessary). CEC, investigator, and CP take appropriate precautions to ensure confidentiality of proceedings. CEC may use tracking sheet developed by JC. CEC Chair advises JC of status of issues before CEC. CEC may stay proceedings if conduct is subject of legal action.

CEC Recommendations
CEC may take one of two actions: dismiss the charges or recommend that JC take one of four disciplinary actions:
(1) Reprimand
(2) Probation for a specified time frame (6 months to 2 years) with corrective action
(3) Suspension of member rights and privileges for not less than 1 year
(4) Expulsion (reinstatement subject to Association bylaws)
CEC notifies the respondent of its recommendations and right to a hearing with the JC (if disciplinary recommendation, transmits the record to the JC, destroys duplicate records, and monitors probationary corrective action).

Decision of the JC
JC makes decision to do one of the following:
Impose the disciplinary action recommended by the CEC and specify effective dates
Impose less severe disciplinary action or dismiss the charges
Remand to CEC with directives
JC notifies respondent of decision and right to appeal to APTA Board of Directors (BOD), notifies CEC of decision, and publishes name of suspended or expelled member in *PT Magazine* and *Physical Therapy*.

Appeal to APTA BOD
Respondent may appeal within 30 days. BOD may make one of the following three decisions:
Affirm JC decision
Modify decision: dismiss charge or impose less severe disciplinary action
Remand to JC with appropriate directives

Figure 3.2 Initiation of disciplinary proceedings (cases not involving criminal offenses). (APTA = American Physical Therapy Association.)

order to initiate the process, Frieda must send the president a written, signed complaint that describes the alleged violation. Frieda addresses a letter to the chapter president stating that she believes that Linda Waller engaged in unethical behavior by advertising her services as a hand specialist when she has no certification in that area. She encloses a copy of the advertisement in the complaint.

On receipt of this letter, the chapter president acknowledges to Frieda receipt of the complaint, enclosing a copy of the *Procedural Document*. The letter to Frieda advises her that Linda Waller has the right to know the identity of the complainant. At the same time, the president forwards a copy of the complaint to the APTA Judicial Committee.

The chapter president must now decide whether the alleged ethical violation is actionable and warrants referral to the CEC—that is, that the alleged conduct, if true, is a violation of the *Code* and the action is not so trivial or so long ago that referral is unwarranted. If determination of the ethical violation involves legal resolution beyond the ability of the CEC, the action may also be deemed unwarranted. In this case, the chapter president decides that the complaint is both actionable and warrants referral.

The chapter president initiates the disciplinary process by the following actions.

1. Notice of the charges is sent to the respondent by certified mail, return receipt requested, within 15 days of determining that the complaint is actionable and warrants referral. This notice must
   a. Fully describe the action
   b. State the portions of the *Code* or *Standards* that have been violated if the complaint is true. It may also allude to possible violations of the *Guide*, but there is no requirement that it do so.
   c. Inform the respondent that the matter is being forwarded to the CEC and provide the name, address, and telephone number of the CEC chair.
   d. Inform the respondent of his or her right to see the complaint.
2. A copy of the notice of charges is sent to the Judicial Committee.
3. A copy of the notice of charges and complaint is sent to the CEC.

Linda Waller receives a letter from the chapter president stating that a complaint has been received. The complaint alleges that Linda has engaged in unethical conduct in that she has advertised her services as a specialist when she is not a certified hand therapist. The letter continues to say that, if this is true, it could constitute a violation of Principle 6 of the *Code* ("Physical therapists provide accurate information to the consumer about the profession and about those services they provide") and, specifically, section 6.2C of the *Guide* ("Physical therapists shall not use, or participate in the use of, any form of communication containing a false, plagiarized, fraudulent, misleading, deceptive, unfair, or sensational statement or claim").

When the investigator appointed by the CEC interviews Linda Waller, Linda tells the investigator that Frieda Findlay's motives are purely financial. "I've been treating hand injuries for decades, and, if that is not a specialty, I do not know what is. Frieda wants my business and she wants to discredit me," Linda said.

QUESTIONS FOR FURTHER REFLECTION

1. As a member of the CEC, what further information would you need to know about this case?

2. Has Linda Waller provided misleading information to the public?

3. How will you sort out possible financial incentives for Frieda's claims? Do these financial motives negate the validity of the claim?

4. Given the limited amount of information provided, what would you recommend to the Judicial Committee?

5. See Table 3.2 for a summary of ethical case resolution during this period. Have you seen misleading advertisements for physical therapy?

6. What are the permissible limits of physical therapy advertising?

7. Does antitrust law, with its focus on free markets and competition, adequately account for the influence of third-party payers?

CASE 3.2

Pat Brooks is a PT in a skilled nursing facility; she has been in practice for 2 years. She is approached with a business proposition by a vendor of orthotic devices. He offers to pay Pat $25 for every orthosis referral she makes to his company. Pat is very uncomfortable with this offer but uncertain what action(s) she should take. She believes that the vendor is a close personal friend of the facility administrator. What legal and ethical issues are raised?

HEALTH CARE FRAUD AND ABUSE

In today's increasingly competitive marketplace, health care entities are aggressively attempting to secure referral sources and optimize reimbursement. Of concern are arrangements that go beyond protection of legitimate business interests and attempt coercive persuasion regarding referrals or that mischaracterize the scope of services provided. The exact cost to taxpayers and consumers of health care fraud and abuse is difficult to pinpoint, but it appears to be significant. One

Table 3.2
American Physical Therapy Association violations and resolutions, 1983–1993

Number	Alleged Violation	Number Dismissed	Informal (No Longer in Effect)	Reprimand	Suspension	Expulsion	Flagged (Membership Expired)
34	Inadequate supervision	9(1)*	7(3)*	14	2	—	2
32	Unprofessional conduct	21	6(1)*	2	—	—	3
19	Misleading advertisements or statements	8(1)*	7	3	—	—	—
9	Excessive fees	9	—	1	—	—	—
11	Fraud (insurance or Medicaid)	1	—	—	4	3	3
9	Unauthorized treatment	3	3	1	1	—	1
6	Documentation	2	—	1	1	—	2
7	Sexual misconduct	2	1	—	1	1	2
5	Felony or battery	—	—	—	1	3	1
4	Overutilization	1	2	1	—	—	—
9	Without valid license	8	—	1	—	—	—
3	Drug or alcohol abuse	1	—	1(1)*	1	—	—
2	Kickbacks	2(2)*	—	—	—	—	—
1	Equipment endorsement	1	—	—	—	—	—
1	Forgery	—	—	—	1	—	—
1	Physician employer	1	—	—	—	—	—
2	Unpaid educational loan	2	—	—	—	—	—
Total 155		71	26	25	12	7	14

*Number of cases with conditions imposed by chapter ethics committee indicated in parentheses.
Source: Adapted from APTA Judicial Committee Report. Ethical Violations/Resolutions 1983–1993. Alexandria, VA: American Physical Therapy Association, 1994.

estimate is that the annual cost of health care fraud and abuse is $100 billion, or approximately 10% of the nation's health care costs.* While this 10% figure is widely quoted, some commentators assert that there is no empirical evidence for the claim and note differences in defining fraud, abuse, and waste.[27] Curbing abuse has become a major emphasis for both state and federal lawmakers seeking to recapture scarce health care dollars. Federal and state enforcement efforts have also intensified since the 1980s. Under the Health Insurance Portability and Accountability Act of 1996, additional funding was granted to combat health care fraud and penalties were increased.[28] From 1987 through the first part of 1995, 1,194 investigations were opened under the anti-kickback law, with more than 716 convictions, settlements and exclusions, and monetary recoveries totaling nearly $25.5 million.† Criminal prosecutions rose from 30 in 1982 to 181 in 1993. Exclusions increased from 230 in 1983 to 881 in 1993. During the same period, civil money penalties cases jumped from six cases (yielding $1.4 million) to 75 cases (yielding $140 million). Most prevalent were cases involving billing for services not rendered, unbundling services, upcoding, kickbacks, and self-referrals.

This scrutiny reflects a heightened public awareness that referral of abuses can have a real impact on cost and quality of care. A 1989 study by the Florida Health Care Cost Containment Board showed that physician-owned physical therapy joint ventures provided 43% more visits per patient than nonphysician-owned services.[29] The report concluded that quality of care in physician-owned clinics was lower than nonphysician-owned clinics and that joint venture facilities did not increase access to services. A 1992 California Worker's Compensation study demonstrated that physicians with an ownership interest in a physical therapy clinic referred 66% of potential patients to the clinic; those without such an interest referred 32%.[30] According to a 1994 report by the Office of the Inspector General (OIG), four of five cases reimbursed as physical therapy in physician's offices do not represent true physical therapy services.[31] The OIG estimated that $47 million was inappropriately paid in 1991 alone for such therapy services (see Chapter 2 regarding delegation issues in this context).

---

*Remarks of Sen. Tom Harkin (D-Iowa) before the Senate Appropriations Subcommittee on Labor, Health and Human Services, Education and Related Agencies, April 22, 1995.

†These figures come from the testimony of Inspector General June Gibbs Brown before the Senate Appropriations Subcommittee on Labor, Health and Human Services, Education and Related Agencies, April 22, 1995. Unbundling refers to charging separately for individual components of a single procedure. Upcoding is charging for a more expensive service than that actually provided; for example, charging for a 30-minute visit while actually providing 15 minutes.

Historical Perspective of Fraud and Abuse

A legal analyst looking at a historical perspective of health care fraud and abuse reviewed 372 legal cases that occurred between 1909 and 1993.[32] The most prevalent forms of abuse, in descending order of frequency, were (1) prescription by fraud; (2) billing for services not performed; (3) misrepresenting the nature of services provided to obtain insurance coverage; (4) auto accident scams (false medical information generated to obtain insurance reimbursement); (5) quackery (inflating curative nature of services); (6) filing false cost reports; (7) soliciting, paying or receiving kickbacks; and (8) providing and billing for unnecessary services.

Statutes and Cases Addressing Fraud and Abuse

Both federal and state statutes address fraud and abuse in the health care environment. However, just what constitutes fraud and abuse in health care is difficult to define. *Fraud* is generally considered misrepresentation of facts, such as billing for services not rendered, altering claim forms to show more services than were actually performed, or submitting claims for noncovered services billed as covered services. *Abuse* is excessive, inappropriate care, including overuse, excessive charges, or submitting claims for services that are not medically necessary.

Federal Statutes and Cases

ANTIKICKBACK LAW.   In 1972, several sections were added to the Social Security Act to combat referral abuses in the Medicare and Medicaid programs. In 1977, these were modified through the Medicare/Medicaid Anti-Fraud and Abuse Amendments. Known as the *antikickback statute*, the act proscribes knowingly and willfully soliciting or receiving any remuneration, directly or indirectly, in return for referring an individual to a person for the furnishing of any item or service for which payment may be made in whole or in part under Medicare or Medicaid. These amendments sought to curb fraudulent overuse, while permitting legitimate business arrangements. Note that both the giver and the recipient of a kickback are liable under the act. Additionally, the act prohibits indirect remuneration; thus, investment interests are also targeted. There is an exception under the "safe harbor" provisions (discussed later in this section) for certain publicly traded companies, subject to several conditions.[33]

Violation of the act may result in monetary penalties or exclusion from the program or both. Under the Health Insurance Portability and Accountability Act of 1996 (HIPAA), the reach of the antikickback statute was broadened to include other federal health care programs, including any program that provides health benefits and is funded in whole or in part (directly or indirectly) by the federal government.[28]

Just what constitutes a kickback? No threshold amount is indicated to define a kickback—rather the statute refers to *any* remuneration. In a Michigan case, a nursing home administrator was found guilty under this statute of accepting alcoholic beverages as kickbacks from pharmacists and PTs in exchange for contracts to provide service to the nursing home residents, many of whom were Medicaid recipients.[34] The payments were based on a percentage of the reimbursed Medicaid payments. A drug supplier who refused to go along with the plan was told that his services were no longer needed. The administrator argued that the amounts were legally insufficient to constitute a kickback (although total amounts were not indicated in the case, he had received approximately $416 per month from one pharmaceutical company). The court did not find this argument persuasive, and penalties were imposed.

In a Georgia home health care case, Apria Healthcare Group, although admitting no wrongdoing, agreed to pay $1.7 million to settle charges that it paid kickbacks to physicians to induce referrals of home care patients.[35]

In response to the far-reaching language of the antikickback statute, certain safe harbor provisions have been enacted, most of which do not apply to physical therapy. One exception is the bona fide employee exception, which permits referrals if the referral recipient is a bona fide employee of the referring entity. Note, however, that such relationships may well violate state law.

FALSE CLAIMS ACT.   It is a felony to knowingly and willfully make or cause to be made any false statement of a material fact in any application for any payment or for use in determining rights to such payment under Medicare or Medicaid.[36] Violations of the False Claims Act are punishable by fines and imprisonment. Examples include billing for services not rendered, misrepresenting services (upcoding), or billing for brand name drugs when over-the-counter or generic equivalents are dispensed.

In a Utah case, a PT received a 5-year exclusion for billing for no-shows.[37] The therapist contended that "he merely did as was told by his superiors, that he was ignorant as to the rules concerning billing for no show patients, and that it was the office manager who decided whether to bill Medicaid."[37] The administrative law judge refused to consider these arguments because the therapist had already pleaded guilty to a state law misdemeanor charge regarding misrepresentation of services; this guilty plea served as the basis for the exclusion.

Horizon/CMS Health Care Corporation reached a $5.8 million settlement with the government regarding overcharges for supplies in its nursing homes.[38] The U.S. attorney asserted that the charges were grossly inflated and that the aggressive billing staff had no medical background and received inadequate supervision from medical personnel.

Hospitals, previously somewhat insulated from investigation, are now under increasing scrutiny. The University of Pennsylvania faculty physician services entered into a $30 million settlement agreement for billing for services actually performed by residents; billing for inpatient consultations at the highest levels of the coding system, without reference to the actual services performed; and for inadequate documentation.[39]

In a case involving a durable medical equipment (DME) vendor, the government failed to show by clear and convincing evidence that the vendor submitted false information with intent to deceive.[40] The vendor had added the words "severe hip/knee involvement," regarding functional deficits to certificates of medical necessity for seat lift chairs prescribed for patients with arthritis. The court, in determining that sanctions were not warranted, noted that the vendor had called physicians to verify the condition in each case before altering the certificates.

HIPAA clarifies the intent standard for imposition of civil penalties.[28] A person violates the act if he or she acts in deliberate ignorance or "reckless disregard" of the truth or falsity of the information. No proof of specific intent to defraud is required. HIPAA also heightens penalties for false claims.

OTHER LAWS.   In addition to antikickback laws, federal law contains several specific health care billing practices provisions. These prohibit charging rates greater than those set by a state plan,[41] repeated violation of the terms of an assignment agreement,[42] and charging for physician services not actually provided by a physician.[43]

Federal law also provides for exclusion from participation in the Medicare and Medicaid programs for a variety of related matters, including conviction of a crime relating to fraud, theft, or financial misconduct relating to general delivery of health care; conviction for obstructing a fraud investigation; revocation or suspension of a health care license based on professional competence, professional performance, or financial integrity; submission of claims in excess of the facility's normal charge; providing health care substantially in excess of the patient's needs or that fails to meet the professionally recognized standard of care; failure to grant immediate access to a facility, records, or documents on reasonable request by HHS, OIG, or other investigators; failure to take corrective action regarding abuses of the prospective payment system; and default on health education loans or scholarships.[44]

Another major federal law to curb referral abuses prohibits physicians from referring Medicare or Medicaid patients to certain entities in which the physician or an immediate family member has an ownership or investment interest or a compensation agreement.[45] Originally applicable to clinical laboratory services only, the Stark prohibition now applies to a variety of additional services, including, but not limited to, physical therapy and occupational therapy services, durable medical equipment, prosthetics and orthotics, home health services, and inpatient and outpatient hospital services. The law, effective January 1, 1995, imposes a penalty of $15,000 if the referring physician knew or should have known that the conduct was illegal. The law permits payments to employees and "in office ancillary services" supervised by a physician.

Other federal laws, not specific to health care, have also been used to fight health care fraud and abuse. These include mail fraud laws, RICO, general fraud laws, criminal conspiracy, and money laundering prohibitions. Under such statutes, a New York PT was sentenced to 27 months in prison and ordered to repay $125,000.[46] The therapist pleaded guilty to conspiracy to commit mail fraud after he billed insurance carriers and the federal government for therapy never performed. He also surrendered his physical therapy license. In Atlanta, a PT was convicted on charges of conspiracy, mail fraud, and wire fraud for billing Medicare and Medicaid for services never provided and for services never ordered.[47, 48] The penalty imposed included a 5-year prison term.

FRAUD ALERTS.   As indicated, federal scrutiny of health care fraud and abuse is increasing. The federal government has launched initiatives in the joint venture, DME, home health, and nursing home areas, issuing fraud alerts that describe perceived areas of abuse and that encourage providers to report observed abuse. The joint venture alert specifically cautions investors against shell DME investments, in which an existing DME company continues to control all aspects of the business.[49] DME companies have also been targeted due to schemes in which vendors contact elderly persons and suggest that they may be in need of medical equipment. Such ventures may become paper mills, providing unnecessary or even dangerous equipment to unwary patients.

Another DME fraud alert related to referral or finders fees to health professionals in a position to direct patients to a particular supplier.[50] The example offered in the alert involves respiratory therapists (RTs), but specifically states that it applies to other allied health professionals as well. In the example, the RTs were paid a fee by home oxygen suppliers for each patient referred. Both therapists and suppliers would be subject to criminal penalties in such a case. In another variation, once the referral was made, the referring therapist was paid for setting up the equipment, providing patient instruction, and monitoring. Were these situations to occur, they would be scrutinized closely by federal investigators to determine whether such services were provided only to patients referred by that therapist, whether therapists were used for patients not referred by them, whether there were any unusual geographic or medical reasons for using therapists in certain cases, and what the area practice is. The bottom line is whether the fee is intended to induce referrals rather than to provide actual services.

The OIG Home Health Care Alert noted that Medicare payments for home health care services have increased significantly since 1990.[51] Federal enforcement officials are specifically looking for claims for visits not made, services provided to beneficiaries that are not homebound or do not require a qualifying service, or services not authorized by a physician. Additionally, "if agency personnel believe that services ordered by a physician are excessive or otherwise inappropriate, the agency cannot avoid liability for filing improper claims simply because a physician has ordered the services."[51]

State Statutes

States have also been involved in the attack on fraud and abuse; there has been a proliferation of state laws to combat fraud, particularly self-referral schemes. Many state legislatures have adopted specific measures to combat health care provider referral fraud and abuse that may restrict professional and business behavior. Others have incorporated fee-splitting provisions within the practice acts. Many states forbid fee splitting, rebates, and kickbacks for referrals through specific referral-for-profit legislation, as well as through the physical therapy practice acts. A few states apply general corporate fraud or bribery statutes to medical service providers. Some state statutes focus on the provider of services, some on the referring professional, and some on both. States differ in application of antifraud statutes; prohibiting direct referrals, indirect referrals, joint ventures, and other contractual arrangements; or any of the above that could imply a kickback. It is important for therapists to be acquainted with the specific restrictions imposed under state law, which may include licensure actions.

Private Insurer Investigations of Fraud and Abuse

In addition to federal and state law enforcement, private insurers are intensifying internal investigations into suspected abuse. According to one survey, investigations by private insurers were up 75% during the early 1990s to 26,755 per year; two-thirds of the cases involve provider fraud.[52] Most common are investigations for fraudulent diagnosis or date of service, billing for services not rendered, and waiver of copayment. Insurers may refuse to pay claims and may also bring such cases to the attention of state and federal authorities for criminal and civil prosecution.

Application to Case 3.2

If Pat elected to participate in the fee-for-referral proposal, she would likely violate federal law regarding kickbacks and referral for profit, subjecting her to criminal and civil penalties. If she falsified patient data to suggest the need for orthoses, she would also be subject to a false claims action. In addition, she might be in violation of state laws specifically designed to curb referral for profit as well as her state practice act.

It is clear that from a legal perspective, Pat would be unwise to participate in this arrangement. This case illustrates again the importance of context and the unique nature of medicine. While these kinds of gratuities are common in other industries, they are considered unethical or illegal in the health care delivery industry. This case illustrates the inherent tension involved in viewing health care as a business.

Pat's acceptance of a kickback could be construed as a violation of the following *Code* principles and *Guide*[21] sections.

Principle 2:   Physical therapists comply with the laws and regulations governing the practice of physical therapy.

Principle 3:   Physical therapists accept responsibility for the exercise of sound judgment.

    3.1C: Regardless of practice setting, physical therapists shall maintain the ability to make independent judgments.

    3.3B: Physical therapists' professional practices and their adherence to ethical principles of the Association shall take preference over business practices. Provisions of services for personal financial gain rather than for the need of the individual receiving the services are unethical.

Principle 5:   Physical therapists seek remuneration for their services that is deserved and reasonable.

    5.1A: Physical therapists shall never place their own financial interest above the welfare of individuals under their care.

    5.3A: Physical therapists shall not use influence upon individuals under their care or their families for utilization of equipment or services based upon the direct or indirect financial interest of the physical therapist in such equipment or services. Realizing that these individuals will normally rely on the physical therapists' advice, their best interest must always be maintained as well as their right of free choice relating to the use of any equipment or service. While it cannot be considered unethical for physical therapists to own or have a financial interest in equipment companies, or services, they must act in accordance with law and make full disclosure of their interest whenever such companies or services become the source of equipment or services for individuals under their care.

5.4A: Physical therapists shall not accept nor offer gifts or other considerations with obligatory considerations attached.

Principle 7:   Physical therapists accept the responsibility to protect the public and the profession from unethical, incompetent, or illegal acts.

7.1B: Physical therapists may not participate in any arrangements in which patients are exploited due to the referring sources enhancing their personal incomes as a result of referring for, prescribing, or recommending physical therapy.

7.2:   The physical therapist shall disclose to the patient if the referring practitioner derives compensation from the provision of physical therapy. The physical therapist shall ensure that the individual has freedom of choice in selecting a provider of physical therapy.

These sections from the *Code* and *Guide* make it clear that Pat's action would be unethical. Presumably Pat could be charged with unethical behavior.

Between 1983 and 1993, the APTA Judicial Committee reported having reviewed the following business-related charges[53]:

- Eleven cases of fraud (insurance/Medicaid)
- Nine cases of excessive fees
- Four overutilization
- Two kickbacks
- One equipment endorsement

QUESTIONS AND NOTES FOR FURTHER REFLECTION

1.   If Pat were to accept this arrangement, should she be subject to disciplinary action? How would this be initiated?

2. Should there be different ethical standards for disclosure of a potential conflict of interest in a business setting as opposed to a medical setting?

3. Vince Longwood is a recent graduate from physical therapy school. He is employed by a large rehabilitation company that maintains contracts to staff skilled nursing facilities. He is often urged to continue treating patients that he does not think have good rehabilitation potential. His bonuses are tied to productivity, and overall census has been low. What legal and ethical dilemmas are posed for Vince? What if the company is owned by a group of referring physicians?

4. Consider the following: an "educational" conference regarding communication devices sponsored by the manufacturer of one device, a PT in private practice who routinely sends gifts to the hand surgeon who refers a significant number of patients; or the PT director who may attend a "free" instruction course (in the Bahamas) if she agrees to purchase an expensive balance evaluation device. Are such "gifts" appropriate? Do they constitute kickbacks?

5. Finley[54] has posed a number of questions therapists should ask themselves in considering the appropriateness of a gift:

    1. Is the gift giving occurring in an effort to express gratitude for services rendered? Is the gift of minimal value?

    2. Is the gift giving an attempt to obligate or control a portion of a PT's practice or research? Are there "strings" attached to receiving the gift?

    3. Is the substance or quantity of the gift(s) large enough to be considered as an issue of kickback?

    4. Is the gift to an institution or organization rather than personal?

    5. Does the gift foster a personal relationship between the professional and the vendor?

    6. Will the gift benefit those in need of our services, or does the professional receive the primary benefit?

    7. Is the cost of the gift ultimately passed on to patients without their knowledge?

    8. Would you be willing to have the gift generally known or disclosed to the patient, the public, or to one's colleagues?

    9. Is the gift of financial support from companies to physical therapists to attend continuing education meetings, for the purpose of

furthering the physical therapy education of the practitioner? Is there reimbursement for essential expenses such as travel, registration, and lodging, rather than personal expenses? Is it a personal pleasure trip with a token educational experience?

EVOLUTION OF THE TRADITIONAL PHYSICIAN-PATIENT RELATIONSHIP: RAMIFICATIONS FOR THE PROVIDER-PATIENT RELATIONSHIP IN A MANAGED CARE ENVIRONMENT

Each principle of the *Code* or section from the *Guide* presumes a trusting relationship between provider and patient in which the primary consideration is the well-being of the patient. One of the foundations of medical ethics is the sanctity of the physician-patient relationship, which dates back to the writings of Hippocrates. With the advent of managed care, medicine is increasingly viewed from a business perspective. How does the shift toward a business perspective affect this relationship?

Defining Managed Care

What is meant by managed care? "*Managed care* describes many different medical care constructs. A managed care organization is one in which specific measures are taken by the provider system or health insurance program to provide health services to a given population within a specific budget."[55] MCOs take a variety of forms, including but not limited to health maintenance organizations (HMOs), preferred provider organizations, physician-hospital associations, and other forms of networks. Such entities vary with respect to the degree of shared risk, the locus of decision-making authority, and assignment of liability. Although this chapter refers to MCOs generally, the reader should be aware that the structure and control mechanisms of the particular organization involved in a given case may affect the legal and ethical analysis applied.

Essentially, managed care refers to any system in which the emphasis is on controlling costs. Common methods of controlling costs in managed care include disincentives, such as the following, to discourage use of health care.

- Copayments for care
- Increased cost for medical care outside the system

- Using primary care physicians as gatekeepers. (Gatekeepers are providers who control access to further services. PTs can serve as gatekeepers in recommending equipment. Although physicians have historically served as gatekeepers, managed care presents a twist to the role. Traditional insurance provided financial incentives to gatekeepers to overutilize health care resources; in contrast, managed care provides possible incentives to underutilize services.)
- Capitation is another method used by MCOs to limit costs. In a capitation arrangement, providers are paid a certain amount per plan member per month to provide all therapy services needed.[56]
- Shift to outpatient services[55]

Rothman[57] is among those who have criticized managed care for bringing these outside influences into the provider-patient relationship. However, others point out that trends of the last 50–75 years represent a multifaceted process of increasing autonomy for the medical profession, increasing costs, involvement of numerous interest groups, and decreasing confidence in the medical professions.[58] More recent emphasis on patients' rights is, therefore, merely a counterbalance to the increasing autonomy of the medical professions. In *Strangers at the Bedside*, Rothman describes the marked increase in the number of persons ("outsiders") involved in patient care. As Rothman points out, this is due in part to the insider-versus-outsider culture that permeates medicine, but it also reflects the increasing involvement of ethics committees, legal entities, third-party payers, and business interests.[57]

The significance of this development is that the relationship between patients and physicians, and indeed all health care providers, has changed. The following section addresses changes in the relationship between providers and patients. (In discussing this topic, the term *provider-patient relationship* is used. Although the literature is oriented to the physician-patient relationship, the insights have important ramifications for other health care providers.)

Provider-Patient Relationship

The provider-patient relationship evolved as one of paternalism, going back to Plato and Hippocrates.[59] As the origins of the term imply, *paternalism* suggests that the provider should look after the interests of the patient much as a parent might. The onus is on the provider to determine the best course of action for the patient. To use the language of medical ethics, the provider operated out of a model of beneficence with little regard for concerns of autonomy. Pushed by the patients' rights movement, the democratization of health care, the concomitant involvement of government, and rising costs,[59] the paternalistic model has met with increasing challenges since the 1970s.

Balint and Shelton[59] described a number of alternatives to the paternalistic model:

- *Libertarian model:* emphasizes autonomy; predominant model since World War II
- *Beneficence-in-trust:* physician makes decision based on understanding grounded in a relationship of mutual trust
- *Accommodation model of Siegler:* emphasizes evolving dynamic model of relationship that balances autonomy and paternalism
- *Psychodynamic model:* developed before emphasis on autonomy; emphasizes the educational role of the provider

In a similar vein, Emanuel and Emanuel[60] described four models of the provider-physician relationship. These four models are compared in Table 3.3 with regard to the goals of interaction, the provider's obligations to the patient, the nature and role of patient's values, the role of provider's values, and the concept of autonomy.

Building on the work of Angell[61] and Brennan,[62] Balint and Shelton suggested that health care providers must develop relationships that help to balance individual and societal demands. "Managed care has been perceived by many as creating an environment that places the physician in a situation of a conflict of interest wherein he or she is expected to accept responsibilities toward society at large as well as fulfill the traditional role of advocate for the individual and particular patient."[59] While Angell[61] described this dilemma as becoming a "double agent," Brennan stated that health care reform must address the community and institutional context in which it is delivered.[59] Decisions about each individual's care affect the ability of society in general to deliver health care to all.

Organization and Accountability in Managed Care

Brennan's communitarian view reinforces Wolf's[63] call for organizational mechanisms of due process and Emanuel's call for accountability in managed care. Ezekiel and Linda Emanuel[64] delineated three major models of accountability: professional, economic, and political. These three models represent the interaction of the following three components:

1. Locus of accountability (the *who* of accountability). May be any number of parties: patients, providers, hospitals, managed care plans, professional associations, employers, payers, government, lawyers, courts.

Table 3.3
Four models of the provider-patient relationship

	Paternalistic	*Informative*	*Interpretive*	*Deliberative*
Other names or designations	Parental, "priestly"	Scientific, engineering, consumer	Counselor	Teacher, friend
Goals of interaction	Provider uses skills to diagnose problem; presents selected information to support recommendation; patient gives assent to procedure	Provider gives patient relevant information that allows patient to select the necessary treatment, which provider then delivers	Interpret patient values to assist patient in selecting treatments that are congruent with theses values	Provider presents information and clarifies "values embodied in the … options"
Provider's obligations	Provider discerns best interest of patient; places patient's interest over provider's; seeks views of others when provider lacks knowledge	Technical expertise; to provide information to facilitate patient control	To provide information and other functions of informative model, plus engage in "joint process of understanding"	To provide information; engage in "moral deliberation" with patient
Nature and role of patient's values	Little role	Assumes patient values are static and well known to patient; plays major role	Patient's values are inchoate and incompletely known to self	Patient's values play major role; provider wants to know patient's values to assist in deliberation
Role of provider's values	Shapes conception of patient need	No role	Not a major role; only role is in helping patient to understand patient identity	Play a role in deliberation and provider may promote health-related values

Table 3.3
(continued)

	Paternalistic	*Informative*	*Interpretive*	*Deliberative*
Concept of autonomy	Patient agrees to provider's making decision	Patient has control over medical decision making	Autonomy as "self-understanding" on the part of the patient	Autonomy as moral self-development
Most appropriate use of model	Emergency situations when time limits patient input	Well-informed patients; dominant model behind informed consent	As in *Informative* but does not assume patients know own values as well	Most appropriate for our time; "shared decision making"

Source: Adapted from EJ Emanuel, L Emanuel. Four models of the physician-patient relationship. JAMA 1992;267:2221–2226.

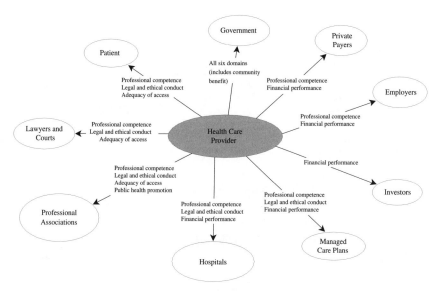

Figure 3.3 Accountability of the health care provider. (Adapted from EJ Emanuel, LL Emanuel. What is accountability in health care? Ann Intern Med 1996;124:229.)

2. Domains of accountability (the *what* of accountability). Generally involves six activities: "professional competence, legal and ethical competence, financial performance, adequacy of access, public health promotion, and community benefit."[60]
3. Procedures of accountability (the *how* of accountability). Figure 3.3 illustrates the loci, domains, and procedures of accountability.

As Emanuel and Emanuel[64] illustrated, accountability is not a simple concept. There are multiple dimensions and types of accountability, including economic, professional, and political accountability.[60] Figure 3.4 illustrates the three major types of accountability. Although calls for increased accountability abound in the managed care environment, it is not clear how that demand might be implemented.

This section addressed the potential impact of MCOs on the provider-patient relationship. The impact of MCOs on patient care outcomes is under study. In an analysis of stroke patients, including 402 HMO patients and 408 fee-for-service patients, Retchin et al.[65] found that HMO patients were less likely to be discharged to rehabilitation hospitals and more likely to be sent to nursing homes after acute care stays. An editorial by Webster and Feinglass[66] suggested that the disparity in rehabilitation referrals is particularly disturbing in light of research in stroke outcomes. They cited a study demonstrating that the

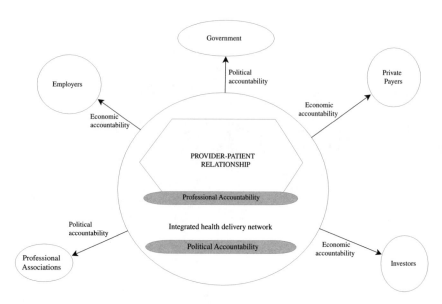

Figure 3.4 Emanuel and Emanuel's "stratified model of accountability."
(Adapted from EJ Emanuel, LL Emanuel. What is accountability in health care?
Ann Intern Med 1996;124:229.)

rate of return to the community for stroke patients treated in rehabilitation hospitals is more than three times the rate of return as compared with patients treated in skilled nursing facilities.

CONFLICTS BETWEEN ETHICS
OF BUSINESS AND MEDICINE

In addition to problems surrounding accountability, there are inherent
conflicts between the traditional ethics of business and the traditional
ethics of medicine. Wendy K. Mariner[67] delineated the problems of
applying traditional ethical standards to MCOs. One major problem in
doing this is that, while traditional medical ethics are directed toward
an individual moral agent, an MCO is not a person. "The organization
is an economic entity, often a corporation—a legal fiction, not a person in a profession with a history of professional ethics. Thus, the ethical principles that have traditionally been thought to apply to health
care practitioners do not easily fit MCOs."[67] Although many organizations fulfill moral functions, appropriate organizational procedures that
delineate appropriate moral standards and measures to ensure due
process have yet to be developed.

Table 3.4

Differences between business and medicine

	Medicine	*Business*
Assumptions about the provider-patient relationship	Trust relationship Unequal knowledge; provider has specialized skill and knowledge	Contractual basis Equal; caveat emptor
Overall goals and purposes	Provide health care services	Efficiency, minimize cost to maximize profit
Ethical principles	Autonomy, beneficence, nonmaleficence; justice (embraces confidentiality, truth-telling)	Fair competition through creation of a fair marketplace in which individuals make voluntary decisions; truthfulness (disclosure); honesty; promise-keeping
Underlying assumption about nature of health care	Service or right	Commodity
Obligation of provider	Fiduciary obligation to patients	Fiduciary obligation to shareholders (for-profit) or to organization or state (nonprofit)

Source: Adapted from WK Mariner. Business versus medical ethics: conflicting standards for managed care. J Law Med Ethics 1995;23:236–246.

To complicate this situation, MCOs must play both a medical and business function. However, as Mariner elaborated, there are significant differences between the assumptions about relationships, ethical principles, and goals of the organization between business and medicine. These differences are summarized in Table 3.4, which is based on her analysis.

Note that one of the primary conflicts is the conflict between maximizing profits and providing for the needs of patients. Although this conflict has been brought into focus by the advent of managed care, it has been an increasing concern since the 1980s. With third-party payers footing the bill for care, providers did not overtly have to choose between quality of care and fiscal accountability because costs (and ethical dilemmas) were hidden. The crisis of escalating costs of Medicare and budget deficits now make it clear that there are ethical dilemmas between providing patient care, fulfilling obligations to stockholders, and acting in the common good. (The argument is that escalating medical costs shift public dollars to health care, thereby decreasing appropriate expenditure on other public goods such as education or roads.) This is implicitly a debate about justice.

What kinds of organizational mechanisms should be enacted to deal with the ethical dilemmas created by managed care? Susan Wolf[63] suggested the following ethical guidelines for organizations.

- Health care organizations should not create financial incentives for physicians to deny patients beneficial treatment.
- Avoiding incentives to deny care is part of a broader obligation to support the capacity of physicians to fulfill their obligations to patients.
- Organizations should establish clear procedures that allow physicians to advocate treatment for individual patients and provide fair initial determination of benefits.
- Organizations should establish fair procedures for patients, surrogates, and health professionals to challenge a denial of benefits.
- Organizations should establish fair processes for monitoring and continuously improving both individual and organizational ethical practice.

Without public policy of this kind, providers will continue to be caught between conflicting obligations to employers and patients. Moreover, patients and the public will have no voice in decisions, nor will they have appeal mechanisms.

CASE 3.3

Peter Santini is a pediatric PT who works in the rehabilitation services department of Mercy Hospital. Mercy Hospital was formerly a nonprofit community hospital, but it has recently been purchased by Gemstone, a for-profit network. When Gemstone purchased Mercy Hospital, many of the employees and townspeople were concerned that they would lose their jobs at the hospital and access to health care. Gemstone has a history of buying and closing hospitals. If Mercy were to close, the nearest hospital would be a 2-hour drive.

Shortly after the purchase, Gemstone eliminated three physical therapy jobs in pediatrics. The company noted that the pediatric area was dependent on Medicaid reimbursement and that rehabilitation services had actually lost money on pediatric physical therapy the preceding year. Peter is now the only pediatric therapist on staff.

Peter's first patient on Monday morning is Paula Holt. Paula is a delightful 3-year-old child who was born with spina bifida.

Peter has been seeing Paula for a little over a year, and she is now nearly ready to walk with a walker. Paula's mother, Sandy, has worked in the cafeteria of Mercy Hospital for 15 years. Sandy is divorced, and her mother takes care of Paula during the day. Although this has been difficult for both Sandy and her mother, Sandy has no other financial resources for day-care for her child.

This morning, it is clear to Peter that Sandy is very upset. "Didn't you get the notice?" she asks Peter. Peter remembers that he did receive something from Gemstone announcing a change in insurance coverage. Sandy tells Peter that the new insurance only allows five physical therapy visits per year. "I just can't afford these bills on my own. Now Paula will never walk."

Peter wonders what he can do about Paula. In his heart, he feels that Paula will be adversely affected by this reimbursement situation.

Is there anything that Peter can do? From an ethical perspective, the case poses the following issues:

1. How should health care be distributed in our society?
2. How can questions of justice in the distribution of health care resources be addressed?
3. What kind of process should be in place to ensure due process when claims are denied?
4. Does Paula have a "right" to a certain level of health care?

The principle of justice is the basis of each of these questions. Although everyone begins early in life to formulate questions about justice, on a conceptual level justice is a complex concept. Fundamentally, the concept of justice requires equal treatment of all people. The duty of justice requires that "similarly situated persons receive their 'fair share' of benefits and assume their fair share of burdens."[68] The problem is to reach some agreement as to what this entails, especially with regard to health care. Justice may be conceptualized as dealing with people equally according to what they deserve or according to merits, or justice may be conceived as dealing with people according to their needs or abilities. A subdivision of the concept of justice is distributive justice. Distributive justice deals with the fair allocation of society's goods and services.[69] Procedural justice refers to fairness of process, which involves due process and an impartial hearing.[68] Managed care faces serious challenges with regard to justice because determination of benefits is linked to cost-saving without public discussion of how benefits should be distributed.

Case 3.3 poses the question of whether Paula has been treated fairly in limiting her care. Without more physical therapy, will Paula have equal access to education and other life experiences? The case also poses the question of which model of justice should be accepted. If everyone receives an equal amount of care, those with more needs may be treated unfairly. Should justice be viewed from the standpoint of needs or from the standpoint of equal allocation of resources?

These concerns regarding justice are superimposed on the societal debate regarding the nature of health care. Is health care a right? Should the market be allowed to determine the distribution of these resources? Society has not reached a consensus on these issues.

In addition to questions of justice, Case 3.3 raises the issue of the responsibility of PTs and PTAs to advocate for the needs of their patients. As previously noted in the discussion of Case 3.2, the *Guide* urges PTs to place the patient's well-being ahead of other considerations. It would, therefore, seem that Peter has an ethical obligation to advocate for his patient.

Section 8.1 of the *Guide* states, "Physical therapists should render pro bono publico (reduced or no fee) services to patients lacking the ability to pay for services, as each physical therapist's practice permits." This suggests that Peter should advocate for his patient and be willing to work out some method of treating his patient, even if Sandy is unable to pay. While this may not be possible in all settings, PTs all too often fail to attempt to work out these kinds of arrangements. The APTA Position on Pro Bono Physical Therapy Services (HOD 86-93-21-39) notes that this responsibility might be discharged by providing services at reduced or no fee, donating professional time to charitable organizations, engaging in activities to improve access to physical therapy, or through financial donations.

As discussed in Chapter 2, society provides freedom to professions in recognition of professions' willingness to police their members. Society places significant trust in professions. In return, members of professions are expected to act in the common good. Pro bono services are a means by which professionals recognize their public responsibility as professionals.

LIABILITY AND ACCESS ISSUES UNDER MANAGED CARE

Access Issues: A Right to Health Care?

Federal health care reform efforts and the advent of managed care have renewed public debate about health care access and the right to health care—an issue raised in Case 3.3. When lawyers speak of rights, they usually are referring to rights accorded under the U.S. Constitution, either explicitly or as interpreted by the courts. Analysis of rights often falls under the fourteenth amendment, which provides (in part) that: "No State shall make or enforce any law which shall abridge the privileges or immunities of citizens of the United States; nor shall any State deprive any person of life, liberty, or property, without due process of law; nor deny to any person within its jurisdiction equal protection of the laws."

These two clauses—the due process clause and the equal protection clause—have generally formed the basis for legal analysis of rights, including the right to health care. Under analysis of these rights, courts have held that all persons have the right to vote, to travel, and to counsel in defense of a criminal charge, but not to health care. As stated by Southwick[70]: "The federal Constitution as interpreted by the Supreme Court does not consider access to health care a fundamental legal right, and denial of non-emergency care based upon an inability to pay for services does not violate principles of constitutional law."

In *Maher v. Roe*,[71] in which several women challenged a Connecticut regulation forbidding state funding for nontherapeutic abortions, the Supreme Court stated: "The Constitution imposes no obligation on the states to pay the pregnancy-related medical expenses of indigent women, or indeed to pay any medical expenses of indigent."

Note that there are certain exceptions when a person is under the control of the state, such as the requirement to provide adequate health care for prisoners.

Congress has adopted several measures to ensure that a minimal societally acceptable level of health care is available to those in need, but there is a distinction between entitlements enacted by Congress, such as Medicare and Medicaid benefits, and Constitutional rights. Congress has chosen to act legislatively to provide benefits for certain individuals, but states are not under a separate Constitutional duty to provide them. Courts have generally given states considerable freedom to circumscribe the boundaries of the health care they do provide, as long as they meet the overarching regulatory requirements of federal programs. Due process is required for state actions that deprive persons of life, liberty, or property. For example, under federal law, due process requirements must be met for Medicaid recipients anticipating service reduction or denials.* Due process mandates reasonable rules that are not unenforceably vague and a fair process, including notice and an opportunity to present information. Increasingly, states are seeking to

---

*42 U.S.C. 1396a(a)(3), requires that the state plan must "provide for a fair hearing before the State agency to any individual whose claim for medical assistance under the plan is denied or not acted upon with reasonable promptness." See also Fair Hearing for Applicants and Recipients, 42 C.F.R. 220; and Establishment of an Expedited Review Process for Medicare Beneficiaries Enrolled in Health Maintenance Organizations, Competitive Medical Plans and Health Care Prepayment Plans, Federal Register 1997 62(83): 23368.

remove themselves from such requirements and to craft their own programs (many using managed care models) for Medicaid recipients under federal block grants by obtaining waivers from traditional Medicaid requirements.

In addition to these two funding programs, under federal law, hospitals cannot refuse to treat patients with emergency medical conditions and women in active labor, regardless of ability to pay.[72] Emergency patients must be medically stabilized before transfer.

Duty to treat may also depend on the hospital's funding or public or charitable status. The Hill-Burton program was enacted during the 1970s to permit additional construction of needed hospital beds.[73] Recipient hospitals of federal Hill-Burton dollars agreed to provide a certain percentage of charitable care. Some plaintiffs have attempted to use this as a defense in collections suits. In *Newsom v. Vanderbilt*,[74] the court determined that the hospital had a duty to provide a reasonable volume of charity care but that the hospital's Hill-Burton obligations did not create a legitimate claim to free services by an individual. Other courts have reached a different conclusion in this matter.[75] Most hospitals, however, have already fulfilled their Hill-Burton obligation.[76] Additionally, some state laws do require government hospitals to provide uncompensated care.

In the private insurance sector, access to health care is largely governed by the insurance contract. Typically, these contracts are negotiated by an individual's employer and provided as a benefit of employment. These vary widely and the contract provisions may be subject to judicial interpretation in the event of a dispute, such as when an insurer seeks to exclude "experimental treatment" to reduce costs.

Without a legal mandate to provide some societally acceptable level of care, how is health care access regulated in a managed care system in which financial incentives to limit service drive medical decision-making? What scope is considered in making such determinations—the needs of a particular patient, of the health insurance plan enrollees, or of society as a whole? Who is to make the determination—the patient, the provider, the insurer, the judge, or the legislature?

Liability in Managed Care

Since the mid-1980s, there have been some attempts to impose liability on MCOs for improper denial of recommended services. The former rule of law had been that such corporations did not control medical judgment; however, some cases have been successful and courts have evinced an increasing willingness to look to the degree of control the company exercises over its physicians and whether a denial of services is a substantial factor in any injury. One early case is *Wick-*

line,[77] involving a patient with arteriosclerosis who underwent an arterial graft procedure. Following surgery, her physicians petitioned Medi-Cal, California's medical assistance program, for an 8-day hospital stay. Medi-Cal representatives denied the request, granting instead a 4-day stay. The patient developed circulatory complications and ultimately underwent an above-the-knee amputation. An initial jury verdict sided with the patient. On appeal, however, the court did not impose liability on Medi-Cal in this case, noting:

> The patient who requires treatment and who is harmed when care which should have been provided is not provided should recover for the injuries suffered from all those responsible for the deprivation of such care, including, when appropriate, health care payors. Third party payors of health care services can be held legally accountable when medically inappropriate decisions result from defects in the design or implementation of cost-containment mechanisms as, for example, when appeals made on a patient's behalf for medical or hospital care are arbitrarily ignored or unreasonably disregarded or overridden. However, the physician who complies without protest with the limitations imposed by a third party payor, when his medical judgment dictates otherwise, cannot avoid his ultimate responsibility for his patient's care. He cannot point to the health care payor as the liability scapegoat when the consequences of his own determinative medical decisions go sour.[77]

Such cases recognize the limits that MCOs may attempt to place on provider decision-making authority and the direct relationship between the MCO and the provider. "HMOs contend that because they do not 'practice' medicine, they are not fiscally liable for the adverse consequences of a bad medical decision. Physicians, on the other hand, feel that HMOs through clinical guidelines or coverage policies are significantly influencing their judgment and thus should be culpable for poor medical outcomes if they are related to a claims payment decision. Most legal health experts will accede that there is a clear trend to make health plans more liable for their decisions in this area."[78]

In a widely publicized case in California ("Jury tells HMO to pay damages in dispute over refused coverage," *Wall Street Journal*, December 28, 1993), an arbitration panel determined that Health Net officials had improperly denied authorization of a bone marrow transplant for a woman with breast cancer.[79, 80] The insurance officials had apparently interfered with the physician's judgment through telephone calls and other communications that the panel concluded constituted "extreme and outrageous behavior exceeding all bounds usually tolerated in a civil society." An $89 million dollar recommendation was made by the panel. This case was later settled out of court for an undisclosed amount.

A number of cases involving bone marrow transplants have been brought, with some judges stretching the limit of contractual liability to provide patients coverage. These cases illustrate the tension between judicial (and provider) desire to give patients what they need as opposed to what they have contracted for or the limits society is able and willing to sustain.[79]

Entities have also been held liable under theories of respondeat superior if the involved physician is an employee,[81] or under an ostensible agency theory if the patient reasonably believes that the physician was acting as the employee or agent of the entity.[82] Other claims may include breach of contract, bad faith breach of contract, fraud, and breach of fiduciary duty.[83] In *Dukes v. U.S. Health Care*,[84] a type of corporate negligence theory was applied. The MCO was charged with failure to adequately select and monitor the performance of its network physicians.

Abandonment

Failure to continue treatment of a patient in need of services may also give rise to a claim of abandonment. *Abandonment,* usually applied to physicians, refers to discharge of a patient in need of medical services without a referral to a suitable alternative care provider. For a patient to recover damages for abandonment, he or she must show that medical care was unreasonably discontinued against the patient's will, that the provider failed to arrange for care by another provider, that it was reasonably foreseeable that harm might occur to the patient because of the termination of care, and that actual harm occurred.[85]

Provider Incentives

Another issue influencing treatment decisions by physicians is provider incentives—that is, bonuses paid to physicians who limit service costs. Effective January 1, 1997, under federal regulation, MCOs that have Medicare risk contracts are prohibited from providing significant incentives to providers to limit or reduce medically necessary treatment provided to individual enrollees.[86] Such referral services include inpatient and outpatient (such as physical therapy) services that are not furnished directly by the referring physician. Incentive structures must be disclosed to enrollees. Additionally, the regulations limit the amount of physician income that may be placed at risk.

Corporate Practice of Medicine Doctrine

A legal theory that has helped insulate medical decision-making from business considerations is the corporate practice of medicine doctrine.

The doctrine provides that a corporation may not practice medicine—that is, physicians are not to be under corporate control because of potential adverse effects on patient care. The doctrine has waned in many jurisdictions but is being explored anew in the face of the increasingly complex corporate-physician relationship in managed care. "Although its enforcement is erratic throughout the U.S., for many the Doctrine has come to symbolize the growing tensions between the traditional values in which twentieth century medical practice was built and the realities it faces in a managed care environment. The Doctrine arose out of fears that corporate involvement in medical practice would hinder physician independence and clinical judgment and commercialize the practice of medicine. The potential result—patient access to needed medical care—could be jeopardized."[78]

Managed Care Contract Issues for Health Care Providers

This section addresses issues that arise in contracts between MCOs and providers. Consideration of a managed care contract, like all major contracts, requires careful attention to detail. Despite standardized contracts, PTs should be aware of their obligations and attempt to negotiate modifications where appropriate. In a contract dispute, courts often do not permit evidence of oral promises made during negotiations. See Appendix for a managed care contract checklist.

Some substantive provisions may be buried in the definitions section, including such key items as what constitutes covered and noncovered physical therapy services (e.g., is the PT contracting to provide specialty services, such as a certified hand specialist provides?). Another key issue is what constitutes medically necessary services and which party determines what is medically necessary.[87] How are emergency services defined?

One type of contract provision (or, more commonly, an "informal" understanding) that MCOs have instituted prohibits health care professionals from discussing treatment options with a patient until the options have been preapproved by the MCO. Treatment alternatives not covered under an enrollee's health plan, therefore, cannot be discussed. A proposed piece of federal legislation that would prohibit such restrictions (known as gag clauses) was defeated in 1996. However, federal officials have warned MCOs in an advisory letter against enforcing such provisions.[88] As stated by HHS Secretary Donna Shalala, "No beneficiary should be denied the information they need to make a sound, informed decision on their treatment. Patients and doctors must have a free exchange of information." President Bill Clinton has since extended the prohibition to Medicaid managed care plans.[89]

Of course payment methodology must be clearly outlined, whether per case, per capita, or in another form. Other reimbursement provisions are called carve outs and stop-loss provisions. *Carve outs* are exceptions to the usual payment method established for particular (typically high cost) services or circumstances. *Stop-loss provisions* protect providers from an unanticipated volume of patients or intensity of service by setting a threshold, beyond which the payment method shifts to standard or discounted charges.

Other key contract areas include indemnification, or hold-harmless, provisions. Providers should also seek assurances of solvency insurance. Duties of the parties, including such things as utilization review and quality improvement, should be expressly outlined. The process to be followed for resolving contract disputes and the terms and conditions for contract termination should be specified.

Employment Retirement Income Security Act

Liability and contract issues may be influenced by the Employment Retirement Income Security Act of 1974 (ERISA). ERISA is a highly technical federal law governing employee benefits. The purpose of the act is to prevent multistate employers from having to have numerous benefits plans to meet each state's requirements. Federal law preempts or cancels any state laws that relate to certain benefits plans. Some MCOs arguably fall under the purview of ERISA, specifically qualified self-insured employer plans that conduct utilization review or an independent reviewer that is treated as a plan fiduciary under ERISA.[90] However, ERISA does not address many health care benefits issues, including insurance standards and liability (medical malpractice laws), which are usually handled for other types of insurance through state law. What does this mean with respect to MCOs? States cannot require that plans offer specific types of services and benefits or impose liability for negligent utilization decisions. The U.S. Supreme Court has reviewed a New York statute that imposes surcharges on patients covered by certain commercial insurers and HMOs and determined that it is not related to benefits plans under ERISA and, therefore, not preempted.[91]

The Supreme Court recently declined to review a case claiming that ERISA preempts a beneficiary's state lawsuit, despite the lack of an available remedy under ERISA.[92] In this case, a husband brought suit seeking damages after his wife's death. The health plan postponed preauthorization of the wife's autologous bone graft for leukemia.

In another case, a couple sued a health plan for damages for the wrongful death of their unborn child and for emotional damages following a miscarriage.[93] The woman's physician had recommended hospitalization for monitoring, but the insurance company would approve only 10 hours per day of home health nursing care. The fetus went into distress (at a time when the nurse was not on duty) and died. The suit was preempted under ERISA although no other remedy was available.

Legislative Initiatives

The Patient Access to Responsible Care Act (PARCA), introduced by Rep. Charlie Norwood (R-GA) and Sen. Alfonse D'Amato (R-NY), proposes patient selection of providers outside the plan, eliminates gag rules, allows access to a significant number of providers, and permits lawsuits now preempted under ERISA.[31, 94] The bill is being supported by the APTA.

In response to perceived abuses in the MCO industry, many states have passed legislation or are considering bills dealing with MCOs. During the first half of 1996, 33 states enacted consumer protection laws related to managed care.[95] Currently, state attempts to regulate MCOs vary widely. Legislative initiatives address utilization review, any willing provider statutes (discussed later in this section), liability issues, and freedom of choice (laws enabling enrollees to self-refer to a non-preferred provider). Additionally, some states have enacted laws mandating coverage for certain types of treatments. Regulatory mechanisms, often through agencies that regulate the insurance industry, also vary from state to state. Credentialing and quality issues may be addressed through regulatory oversight.[96]

Some state statutes, known as *any willing provider (AWP) laws*, require MCOs to use any provider that meets certain standards. Some of the pros and cons of AWP laws are shown in Table 3.5. The AWP issue is not just a hypothetical situation for PTs. On July 28, 1995, the Arkansas AWP law became effective. The state chapter had joined a coalition to promote the law. Several insurers have successfully challenged the law on grounds that the law is preempted by ERISA.[97] Courts that have considered the ERISA issue with respect to AWP laws are split, and the Supreme Court has denied petitions for certiorari in this area. New state initiatives tend to focus on antigag clause provisions, physician financial incentive disclosure, utilization review criteria, definitions of emergency situations, and clinical practice guidelines.[95]

Although the legal implications and liability issues that arise in managed care have yet to be settled, it is clear that a significant number of insurance beneficiaries are covered by MCOs and that the number is likely to grow. According to a survey of 2,037 employers conducted by KPMG Peat Marwick and Wayne State University researchers, nearly

Table 3.5
Pros and cons of any willing provider laws

Pros	Cons
Promote equity among providers; open markets	Decrease administrative efficiency for MCO of limited number of contracts and providers
Serve the best interests of patients because free choice is permitted; raise standards through competition; may decrease travel distance	May decrease incentives to participate based on volume because use of capitation method of billing is difficult, if not impossible
Allow providers to select MCO with proven track record	Do not permit MCOs to select providers with proven track record

MCO = managed care organization.

three-fourths of U.S. workers with health insurance were in some form of managed care by 1995, a 50% increase since 1993.[98]

Application to Case 3.3

Case 3.3 states that Sandy's insurance will cover only five PT visits per year for Paula. However, many questions are left open. Is this a new contract provision? Has there been a change in interpreting an existing policy? On what basis? Does the insurance company provide for an appeals process? What duty does Peter have to contact the insurer, to submit a request for reconsideration, or to appeal the determination? The *Wickline* case suggests that health care providers owe a duty to patients to appeal treatment denials that they believe to be in error. Thus, Peter should, at a minimum, investigate options regarding the denial. If a state insurance mandate covering such care exists, Sandy may have legal recourse to compel treatment.

QUESTIONS AND NOTES FOR FURTHER REFLECTION

1. Is there a minimally acceptable level of health care to be provided to all persons? Whose interests should be taken into account in determining the proper level of care for an individual?

2. For a discussion of legal issues related to managed care, refer to *Legal Answer Book for Managed Care.*[99]

3. How should society resolve the conflict between business ethics and traditional medical ethics inherent in managed care?

4. What measures should an MCO institute to establish account-ability and provide due process for consumers?

5. What are the ethical dilemmas encountered by PTs as gate-keepers in fee-for-service and in managed care environments?

6. Under what circumstances should PTs provide pro bono ser-vices? What are some ways to accomplish this within organiza-tional constraints in your setting?

7. See generally Martin and Bjerknes.[100]

8. For a discussion on managed care, see the July 1993 issue of *PT Magazine*.

REFERENCES

1. *American Medical Assn. v. Federal Trade Commission*, 638 F.2d 443 (2nd Cir. 1980).
2. *Virginia State Board of Pharmacy v. Virginia Citizens Consumer Council, Inc.*, 425 U.S. 748 (1976).
3. *Ohralik v. Ohio State Bar*, 436 U.S. 447, 462 (1978).
4. 15 U.S.C.A. §41-58.
5. Statement of Policy Regarding Comparative Advertising, 16 C.F.R. §14.15.
6. 15 U.S.C. §45(l) and 45(m)(1).
7. 15 U.S.C. §1125(a).
8. Edelstein J (ed). Challenging False Advertising by a Competitor: The Options—Their Pros and Cons. In False Advertising and the Law. New York: Practising Law Institute, 1996;7.
9. Scott R. Advertising PT services: legal implications. PT Mag 1993;1:55.
10. Schunk C, Hruska R. Physical therapy and advertising. PT Mag 1993;1:52.
11. Hawaii Revised Statutes Annot., Chapter 461J-12(a)(3) and (4).
12. 15 U.S.C.A. §1-7.
13. 15 U.S.C.A. §12-27, 44.
14. 15 U.S.C. §45(a)(1).
15. *Hospital Corp of America v. FTC*, 807 F.2d 1381 (7th Cir. 1986).
16. Statement of antitrust enforcement policy in health care. BNA Health Law Reporter August 28, 1996;5:1306.
17. *Wilk v. American Medical Association*, 895 F.2d 352 (7th Cir. 1990).
18. *American Medical Assn. v. U.S.*, 317 U.S. 519 (1942).
19. *New York State Chiropractic Association*, D. 9210 (FTC consent order issued Nov. 11, 1988, 53 *Federal Register* 52,405.)
20. American Physical Therapy Association. House of Delegates Policies. Alexan-dria, VA: American Physical Therapy Association, November 1996;i.
21. APTA Guide for Professional Conduct. Alexandria, VA: American Physical Therapy Association, 1997.
22. Beauchamp TL, Childress JF. Principles of Biomedical Ethics (4th ed). New York: Oxford University Press, 1994;38, 483.
23. American Physical Therapy Association. Standards of Practice for Physical

Therapy and the Clinical Accompanying Criteria. Alexandria, VA: American Physical Therapy Association, 1995.

24. American Physical Therapy Association. Procedural Document on Disciplinary Action. Alexandria, VA: American Physical Therapy Association, 1996.

25. American Physical Therapy Association. Compendium of Interpretations and Opinions. Alexandria, VA: Judicial Committee of the American Physical Therapy Association, 1995.

26. American Physical Therapy Association. Investigation Guidelines for Chapter Ethics Committees of the American Physical Therapy Association. Alexandria, VA: Judicial Committee of the American Physical Therapy Association, 1995.

27. Mashaw J, Marmor T. Conceptualizing, estimating and reforming fraud, waste and abuse in health care spending. Yale J Regulation 1994;11:455.

28. Health Insurance Portability and Accountability Act of 1996, Pub. L. 104-191, HR 3103.

29. Mitchell J, Scott E. Physician ownership of physical therapy services—effects on charges, utilization, profits, and service characteristics. JAMA 1992;268:2055.

30. Swedlow A, Johnson G, Smithline N, et al. Increased costs and rates of use in the California worker's compensation system as a result of self-referral by physicians. N Engl J Med 1992;327:1502.

31. Ellis J. Physical therapists storm the Hill to educate legislators about PT profession. PT Bull 1997;12:10.

32. Bucy, P. The poor fit of traditional evidentiary doctrine and sophisticated crime: an empirical analysis of health care fraud prosecutions. Fordham Law Review 1994;63:391.

33. Program Integrity Medicare and State Health Care Programs, Exceptions. 42 C.F.R. §1001.952.

34. *United States v. Perlstein*, 632 F.2d 661 (1980).

35. Health Lawyers News 1997;1(1):29.

36. 42 U.S.C. §1320a-7(b); 31 U.S.C. §3279.

37. *Dow v. Inspector General*, Doc. No. C-92-061, Dec. No. CR222, Aug. 7, 1992 (Dept. of Health and Human Services Departmental Appeals Board, Civil Remedies Division).

38. Health Lawyers News 1997;1(2):21.

39. *United States v. Clinical Practices of the University of Pennsylvania* (E.D.Pa. Dec. 12, 1995).

40. *United States v. Stelweck*, 108 B.R. 488 (E.D.Pa. 1989).

41. 42 U.S.C. §1320a7b(d).

42. 42 U.S.C. §1320a7b(e).

43. 42 U.S.C. §1320a7b(a)(5).

44. 42 U.S.C. §1320a-7(b).

45. 42 U.S.C. §1395nn.

46. Physical therapist sentenced for billing fraud. PT Bull, November 3, 1993;4.

47. Federal grand jury returns indictment against therapist. PT Bull 1994;9:2.

48. PT arrested in fraud charges. PT Bull, March 30, 1994;3.

49. OIG Special Fraud Alert, Announcement OIG 89-4. CCH Medicare and Medicaid Guide, paragraph 38,448, 1989.

50. Program Memo (Carriers) B-85-2. CCH Medicare and Medicaid Guide 1995; paragraph 13921.71.

51. OIG Fraud Alert, Federal Register 1995;60(154):40847.

52. Health Insurance Association of America. Physicians are leading targets of increasing fraud investigations. PT Bull August 11, 1993;1.

53. American Physical Therapy Association. APTA Judicial Committee Report. Ethical Violations/Resolutions 1983–1993. Alexandria, VA: American Physical Therapy Association, 1994;1488.

54. Finley C. Gift-giving or influence peddling: can you tell the difference? Phys Ther 1994;74:143.

55. Caughey A, Sabin J. Managed Care. In D Calkins, RJ Fernandopulle, BS Marino (eds), Health Care Policy. Cambridge, MA: Blackwell, 1995;88.

56. Ketter P. Understanding driving forces behind managed care is critical for survival. PT Bull 1997;12:6.

57. Rothman DJ. Strangers at the Bedside: A History of How Law and Bioethics Transformed Medical Decision-Making. New York: Basic Books, 1991;2.

58. Starr P. The Social Transformation of American Medicine. New York: Basic Books, 1982.

59. Balint J, Shelton W. Regaining the initiative: forging a new model of the patient-physician relationship. JAMA 1996;275:887, 889.

60. Emanuel EJ, Emanuel LL. Four models of the physician-patient relationship. JAMA 1992;267:2221.

61. Angell M. The doctor as double agent. Kennedy Inst Ethics J 1993;3:279–286.

62. Brennan TA. An ethical perspective on health care insurance reform. Am J Law Med 1993;19:37.

63. Wolf SM. Health care reform and the future of physician ethics. Hastings Center Report 1994;24:28–41.

64. Emanuel EJ, Emanuel LL. What is accountability in health care? Ann Intern Med 1996;124:229–239.

65. Retchin S, Brown R, Yeh S, et al. Outcomes of stroke patients in Medicare fee for service and managed care. JAMA 1997;278:119.

66. Webster J, Feinglass J. Stroke patients, "managed care," and distributive justice. JAMA 1997;278:161.

67. Mariner WK. Business versus medical ethics: conflicting standards for managed care. J Law Med Ethics 1995;23:236–246.

68. Purtilo R. Ethical Dimensions in the Health Professions (2nd ed). Philadelphia: Saunders, 1993;22, 23.

69. Frankena WK. Ethics (2nd ed). Englewood Cliffs, NJ: Prentice-Hall, 1973;48–50.

70. Southwick AF. The Law of Hospital and Health Care Administration (2nd ed). Ann Arbor, MI: Health Administration Press, 1988;290.

71. *Maher v. Roe*, 432 U.S. 464 (1977).

72. Emergency Treatment and Active Labor Act, 42 U.S.C. §1395dd.

73. 42 U.S.C. §291c(e)(2).

74. *Newsom v. Vanderbilt*, 653 F.2d 1100 (1981).

75. *Creditors Protective Ass'n, Inc. v. Flack*, 763 P.2d 756 (1988).

76. Miller R. Problems in Health Care Law (7th ed). Gaithersberg, MD: Aspen, 1996;95.

77. *Wickline v. State of California*, 192 Cal. App. 3d 1630, 239 Cal. Rptr. 810 (1986).

78. National Health Lawyers Association and the American Academy of Healthcare Attorneys. Patient Care and Professional Responsibility: Impact of the Corporate Practice of Medicine Doctrine and Related Laws and Regulations. Washington, DC: National Health Lawyers Association and the American Academy of Healthcare Attorneys, 1997.

79. Morreim H. Moral justice and legal justice in managed care: the ascent of contributive justice. J Law Med Ethics 1995;23:247.
80. Meyer M, Murr, A. Not my health care. Newsweek 1994;123(2):36.
81. *Sloan v. Metropolitan Health Council*, 516 NE2d 1104 (Ind. Ct. App. 1987).
82. *Gilbert v. Sycamore Municipal Hospital*, 622 NE2d 788 (Ill. 1993).
83. *Gross v. Prudential Health Care Plan*, No. CJ-9474267 (Okla. Cty. Ct. Oct. 1, 1996).
84. *Dukes v. U.S. Health Care*, 57 F.3d 350 (3d Cir. 1995).
85. Pozgar GD. Legal Aspects of Health Care Administration (5th ed). Gaithersburg, MD: Aspen, 1993.
86. Medicare and Medicaid programs; requirements for physician incentive plans in prepaid health care organizations. 61 Federal Register 1996:13;430; as amended 61 Federal Register September 3, 1996: 46,384, 61 Federal Register 69034 (Dec. 31, 1996).
87. Banghart S. Managed care contract checklist. PT Mag July, 1993;26.
88. Government changes rules for HMOs enrolling Medicare, Medicaid recipients. PT Bull January 10, 1997;1.
89. Health Lawyers News 1997;1(3):7.
90. 29 U.S.C. 7144(a).
91. *New York State Conference of Blue Cross Blue Shield Plans v. Travelers Ins. Co.*, 115 S.Ct. 1671, 131 L.Ed. 2d 695 (1995).
92. *Cannon v. Group Health Serv. of Okla., Inc.*, 77 F.3d 1270, No. 95-1927, cert. denied, 65 U.S.L.W. 3257 (U.S. Oct. 7, 1996).
93. *Corcoran v. United Healthcare Inc.*, 965 F.2d 1321 (5th Cir. 1992).
94. New managed care reform bill would put patients ahead of profits. PT Bull 1997;12:1.
95. Managed care consumer protection laws enacted in more than 30 states. PT Bull 1996;11(31):1.
96. Gosfield A. Who is holding whom accountable for quality? Health Affairs 1997;16:26.
97. *Prudential Insurance Co. v. National Park Medical Center Inc.*, Health Lawyers News 1997;1(3):21.
98. Jensen G, Morrisey M, Gaffney S, Liston D. The new dominance of managed care: insurance trends in the 1990s. Health Affairs 1997;16:125.
99. Younger P, Connor C, Aspen House Law Center Staff. Legal Answer Book for Managed Care. Gaithersburg, MD: Aspen, 1995.
100. Martin J, Bjerknes L. The legal and ethical implications of gag clauses in physician contracts. Am J Law Med 1996;22:433.

Appendix

Managed Care Contract List

1. **Parties**
   ___ Are the parties clearly identified?
   HMO: Does the contract cover—
   ___ Whether HMO is licensed and federally qualified?
   ___ Multiple benefit plans?
   ___ Relationship with a PPO/insurance company?
   ___ HMO's stability, financial and otherwise?
   PPO: Does the contract specify—
   ___ Whether PPO is insured? Incentivized?
   ___ Is the correct contracting entity identified?
   ___ Are all parties with obligations under the contract either included or made third-party beneficiaries?

2. **Preface**
   ___ Are the recitals consistent with the terms of the contract?
   ___ Do the recitals contain only statements that are separately represented, or are the statements found in the body of the contract?

3. **Definitions: Are terms—**
   ___ Used consistently throughout the contract?
   ___ Clearly defined?
   ___ Are specific definitions included?
   ___ Emergency admission, and who makes that determination
   ___ Medical necessity
   ___ Elective admission
   ___ Urgent admission
   ___ Covered and noncovered services
   ___ Plan contract or agreement
   ___ Participating physician
   ___ Provider
   ___ Participating hospital
   ___ "Covered person" (i.e., benefit eligibility)
   ___ Payer/contractor
   ___ Claims administrator
   ___ Concurrent review
   ___ Preadmission certification
   ___ Retrospective review
   ___ Case management
   ___ Utilization review administrator

4. **Provider Duties:**
   Does contract specify that provider—
   ___ Ensures licensing consistent with services provided?
   ___ Has the right to refuse to treat patients who are disorderly or problematic?
   ___ Provides verification of eligibility procedure?
   ___ Submits billing in acceptable form?
   ___ Participates in utilization review/quality assurance programs?
   ___ Participates in grievance procedures?
   ___ Makes referrals to other network providers?
   ___ Maintains general/professional liability insurance?
   For example, is provider:
   ___ required only to provide coverage equal to the normal level in the provider's geographic area?

HMO = health maintenance organization; PPO = preferred provider organization.
Source: Reprinted with permission from S Banghart. Managed care contract checklist. PT Mag 1993;1:26.

___ required to name the payer/contractor as an additional named insured?

___ required to provide a certificate of coverage to the payer/contractor?

___ required to provide coverage after termination?

___ required to select insurance carrier subject to payer contractor approval?

___ Meets indemnification requirement?

___ Has patient referral limitations?

___ Obtains prior approval for specified service?

___ Maintains medical records?

___ Provides reasonable access to records?

___ Collects copayment/deductible or coinsurance amounts from covered person?

___ Meets data/reporting requirement?

5. **Payer/Contractor Duties:**
Does contract specify that payer/contractor—

___ Obtains state licensure/certification, if appropriate?

___ Establishes procedure for verification of eligibility?

___ Participates in utilization review?

___ Provides coordination of benefits?
Does contract specify—

___ extent of provider's involvement in coordination of benefit efforts?

___ whether contractor/payer is ultimately liable to provider?

___ Establishes the grievance procedure?

___ Does the marketing (use of provider name controlled)?

___ Must give provider notice of new contracts?

___ Obtains professional and general liability insurance?

___ Meets the indemnification requirement?

___ Reports to provider?

___ Identifies the covered person?

___ Informs covered persons of utilization review obligations and decisions?

___ Collects prescribed fees from covered persons?

___ Administers manual/polices/procedures/benefit plan descriptions?

___ Provides copies of any routine and special reports that may be required by the state departments of health or insurance?

___ Maintains solvency insurance?

___ Provides incentive (financial or other) that will induce covered persons to utilize network providers?

6. **Utilization Review:**
Does contract specify—

___ Clear definitions of duties and costs?

___ Specific standards for utilization review determinations?

___ Appeal procedures and provider's rights and responsibilities in the appeal process?

___ Retroactive denial of payment for physician-ordered services?

___ Payment available for costs related to utilization review participation?

___ Liability issues? For example:

___ Is the care determination process designed to minimize liability?

___ Does the provider receive indemnification for participation in utilization review activities?

___ Quality assurance issues? For example:

___ What is involved in cooperating in a payer/contractor utilization review/quality assurance program?

___ What are the provider's role and responsibilities in the utilization review/quality assurance program?

___ Preadmission review issues? For example:

___ Is there good-faith effort at precertification, meaning diagnosis warrants admission (if required)?

___ Are claim payments based on medical necessity (not precertification)?

___ Is there access to a qualified plan representative 24 hours per day, 7 days per week?

___ Does the precertification process provide authorized length of stay?

___ Is precertification the responsibility of the patient and/or attending physician?

___ Concurrent review issues (restricted to cases not precertified or when length of stay is exceeding that authorized in the precertification process)? For example:

___ Is there on-site review by an outside entity?

___ Is there information provided by telephone or facsimile using appropriate criteria?

___ Is there a fee for review?

___ Is there a limitation on who will perform case management?

___ Is the payer responsible for informing the patient of denial?

___ Retrospective review issues (restricted to cases that have not been precertified or reviewed concurrently)? For example:

___ Are copies available at nominal charge?

___ Is payment based on medical necessity?

___ Is payment not to be withheld pending outcome of review?

___ Whether changes in utilization review and quality assurance program should require at least 30 days written notice with provision for rejection?

7. Claims Management:
Does contract specify—

___ Prompt payment provisions (24 days or less)?

___ Late payment penalty?

___ Periodic interim benefits?

___ An ability to bill the patient if payments have not been received from insurer within "x" number of days?

___ A transmittal format for remittance as specified by provider?

___ No claims filing limit (acceptable filing is within 1 year of service)?

___ Coordination of benefits/subrogation?

___ An automatic assignment of benefits from covered persons to provider?

8. Medical Records:
Does contract specify—

___ Maintenance as required by law?

___ Whether payer/contractor obtains written patient authorization for release of records?

___ Whether payer/contractor pays copy costs?

___ Whether payer/contractor has access in accordance with law?

___ Whether access to data is provided only when necessary?

9. Provider Compensation:
Does contract specify—

___ Payment methodology, such as:

___ capitation?

___ discount on billed charges?

___ per case?

___ risk-sharing?

___ Timeframe?

___ Whether it is the provider's right to bill members for copayments, deductibles, and noncovered services?

___ A clear definition for the methodology of renegotiating rates?

___ Audit opportunities?

___ An acceptable claims turnaround time?

___ Penalties for failure to pay claims in agreed time? For example:

___ Is there an interest charge on an unpaid balance?

___ Does the payer revert to paying the provider's actual charges?

___ Billing forms?

___ A payment appeals process?

___ Risk of nonpayment? For example:

___ Is there a right to bill patient?

___ Is there a limit on responsibility to provide services?

___ Is there a right to receive charges actually made?

10. Patient Duties:
Does contract specify—

___ Whether there are noncovered services (contract should specify liability of patient for noncovered services)?

___ Copayments? For example:

___ How complex are the copayment calculations?

___ Does the provider collect copayments at time of service?

11. Liability Issues:
Does contract specify—

___ Whether liability exposure extends unnecessarily beyond that level to which provider is already exposed?

___ If provider chooses to indemnify payer/contractor, whether the scope of that indemnification is limited to those events and individuals over which provider has reasonable control and whether such indemnification also will be reciprocal in nature?

12. Quality Issues:
Does contract specify—

___ Whether the payer/contractor's quality control procedures conflict with those of the provider?

___ Provider's and payer/contractor's responsibilities in a meaningful way?

13. Marketing:
Does contract specify whether—

___ Payer/contractor's ability to use the name of the provider in description of services is structured to avoid embarrassing provider?

___ Such a description also is structured to eliminate any exposure to unnecessary liability?

14. Insolvency Protection:
Does contract specify whether—
___ Provider will be notified if the payer/contractor receives a special audit or is questioned by the state upon submission of any required report?

15. Term:
Does contract specify—
___ Effective date of contract?
___ Length of term of contract?
___ Procedure and notice period of renewals, if any?
   ___ Does contract require affirmative action to either terminate or renew the agreement?
   ___ Does the contract specify automatic rate increases at renewal?
   ___ Does the contract tie renewal rate increases to an index?

16. Termination:
Does contract—
___ Cover termination without cause?
___ Specify whether there is a remedy period for termination without cause?
___ Specifically state reasons for termination without cause?
___ Specify the ability of provider to quickly terminate contract if payer/contractor stops making payment in timely fashion?
___ Specify rights and duties upon termination, such as:
   ___ Provider's right to be compensated at agreed charge after termination/bankruptcy of payer/contractor?
   ___ Extent of provider's obligation to continue care after termination?
   ___ Survival of important terms after termination (e.g., confidentiality, indemnification, insurance medical records)?

17. Exclusivity:
Does contract specify whether—
___ Exclusivity is limited versus unlimited?
___ *Exclusivity is reviewed by counsel in light of antitrust issues?*

18. General Provisions:
Does contract specify—
___ No amendment or assignment without written approval?
___ Arbitration of dispute and cost recovery, if so desired?
___ Recovery of attorneys' fees and disputes?
___ Binding effect of agreement?
___ Choice of law favorable to provider?
___ Whether agreement is to be held confidential by all parties?
___ Whether agreement constitutes the entire agreement between all the parties?
___ Whether any identification of other contract providers is necessary?
___ Independent contractor status of the parties?
___ Procedure necessary for giving notice?
___ Any reinsurance provisions, as applicable?
___ Whether lack of performance due to unforeseen circumstances is allowed in a limited fashion?
___ No waiver of breach?
___ Whether there are any blank spaces?
___ Whether provisions are separable?
___ Whether signature block is present and accurate?
___ Whether subscription certificates (plan design) are attached as exhibits?
___ Whether all exhibits incorporated by reference are in the agreement?

4

Administrative and Organizational Issues

This chapter focuses on a variety of issues that may be encountered by a physical therapy administrator; these are illustrative and by no means exhaustive. The chapter begins with a case that involves suspected abuse of an elderly patient. Employment issues are then addressed, including an analysis of the Rehabilitation Act, the Americans with Disabilities Act (ADA), and sexual harassment laws. Discussion of risk management principles, using physical therapist (PT) sexual misconduct as a potential departmental risk, concludes the chapter.

Some secondary themes of this chapter are gender relationships and power issues. In some cases, such as domestic violence and relationships between providers and clients, these issues come together. Issues of gender, like those of race, cut across virtually all spheres of medical practice. Some authorities view domestic violence against women as a result of extreme manifestations of sex role stereotypes whereby women are trapped by their passivity. Cases 4.2 and 4.3 deal with relationships of power and gender: sexual harassment in the workplace and dating a client.

CASE 4.1

Elaine Truscott is a home health physical therapy assistant (PTA) in a small rural community. Frieda Simms is a 70-year-old woman whom Elaine has been treating for weakness following a cerebrovascular accident. Elaine suspects that Frieda's son-in-law, Dawson, is physically abusive to Frieda. Dawson is well known in town for his bad temper and violent nature. During physical therapy one morning, Elaine notices bruises all over Frieda's arms. When Elaine asks Frieda about the bruises, Frieda does not answer directly but says, "Dawson has his problems, but at least he gives me and my daughter a place to stay and something to eat. What else can I do?" What should Elaine (and her supervisor) do? Suppose that the patient has asked Elaine not to disclose this information. Suppose that Elaine lives in a state with a mandatory abuse reporting law.

LEGAL ANALYSIS: ELDER ABUSE

Definition and Incidence

Abuse of individuals by others in the home environment poses serious health consequences and is a situation that is sometimes encountered by PTs, although it has not received a great deal of attention in the professional literature.[1] This section highlights elder abuse as one form of domestic abuse that is often overlooked. Of course, child abuse and other types of domestic violence also raise issues regarding the responsibility of health care providers who discover or suspect the abuse.

Definitions of elder abuse vary among state statutes and among authors. All include physical violence, and many include psychological or emotional abuse, material exploitation, and neglect. The issue of whether to include self-neglect within the definition of abuse has not been settled. The following example illustrates how Tennessee has statutorily defined abuse:

(1) "Abuse or neglect" means the infliction of physical pain, injury, or mental anguish, or the deprivation of services by a caretaker which are necessary to maintain the health and welfare of an adult or a situation in which an adult is unable to provide or obtain the services which are necessary to maintain that person's health or welfare.

(8) "Exploitation" means the improper use by a caretaker of funds which have been paid by a governmental agency to an adult or to the caretaker for the use or care of the adult.[2]

Incidence reports of elder abuse vary from approximately 1 to 10 percent of the nation's elderly, depending on how elder is defined and which definition of abuse is used. One researcher,[3] extrapolating from actual reports to state agencies, estimated that the actual number of cases of elder abuse in domestic settings for 1991 was 735,000. The number of estimated cases of self-neglect for 1991 was 842,000. Many elders experience repeated acts of abuse. One study showed that 62% of professionals who deal with the elderly in the community reported seeing indications of physical abuse, and an even higher percent reported experience with other forms of abuse.[4] Pillemer and Moore found that 36% of workers in nursing homes had seen at least one act of physical abuse in the last year; 81% had witnessed psychological abuse such as yelling or insults.[5] Ten percent admitted that they had physically abused a resident themselves; 40% admitted to psychological abuse.

The breakdown of types of abuse varies by definition. A study by Benton[6] suggested the following breakdown: 38% neglect, 28% physical abuse, 20% financial abuse, 11% psychological abuse. Another study by Tatara[3] yielded the following results: 45% neglect, 19% physical abuse, 17% financial abuse, and 14% psychological abuse.

The national trend is toward an increase in reported cases, despite the phenomenon of underreporting. As one research team wrote, "Virtually all state agencies charged with the identification, investigation, and prevention of abuse of the elderly report increases in their caseloads over the past decade."[7] Tatara[3] reported a 94% increase in the number of reports of elder abuse submitted to state agencies from 1986 to 1991. Underreporting is prevalent because the abuse occurs in private homes, families tend to be secretive about abuse, elders themselves are reluctant to report abuse, and there is a lack of professional and public awareness.

A special issue for hospitals is that of abandonment—incidents in which an elderly patient is taken to the emergency room and is unable to be discharged because the family or caretaker has left, the institution from which the patient came refuses to take the patient back, or the patient is alone with no one to care for him or her. A survey by the American College of Emergency Physicians suggested that approximately 70,000 patients were abandoned in 1991 alone.[8]

Several risk factors specific to elder abuse have been identified, and PTs should be familiar with them. These include frailty, cognitive impairment of the victim, shared living arrangement with the abuser, and dependence (usually financial) of the abuser on the elderly person.[7] The American Medical Association (AMA) classifies as high risk elderly individuals who live at home and whose needs exceed or will soon exceed the families' ability to meet them, whose primary caretakers are expressing frustration and signs of stress regarding caretaking responsibilities, and for whom there is a family norm of violence, alcohol, or drug use.[9] One researcher found that the single criterion most predictive of readmission to the hospital was caregiver stress.[10]

There are several unique features of elder abuse, as distinguished from other forms of domestic violence. First, the caregivers themselves may be elderly. There are frequently few options for alternative care providers, such as adult day-care or respite care programs. The abuser may be the only remaining family member, and the elder may fear alternative placement options, such as extended care. Furthermore, fear of discovery of the abuse may discourage elders and their family members from seeking needed medical care.

Although 90–95% of domestic violence in general is committed against women,[11] elder abuse seems to affect men and women more equally. The Canadian Task Force on the Periodic Health Examination[12] noted the following in describing a study by Podnieks of Canadian elderly.

> For material abuse, men and women were equally likely to be victims, the victims tended to live alone, and the perpetrators tended to be distant relatives or nonrelatives. Long-term verbal abuse tended to occur between spouses, with men and women equally affected. Victims of such abuse generally functioned independently but tended to blame themselves. Physical violence was most likely to occur between spouses. Men were more likely than women to be victims, but the violence perpetrated by men tended to be more severe than that inflicted by women.

Although approximately one-fifth of women are estimated to be the victims of domestic violence during their lifetimes,[11] the prevalence of elder abuse is estimated to be between 4 and 10%.[12]

Legal Intervention

At the federal level, Chapter 3 of Title VII of the Older Americans Act provides for public education regarding elder abuse and an ombudsman program.[13] Many states have mandatory or voluntary reporting laws.* The mandatory laws require certain classes of individuals (such as health care workers) or anyone with reason to suspect abuse is occurring to report information to the appropriate state authority. Failure to report can result in criminal penalties.† At least one state court has imposed liability on a physician for failure to report a case of child abuse, under a medical malpractice theory.[14] Some states have adopted specific civil and criminal penalties for elder abuse. For example, under a Texas state statute, it is a felony for a caretaker to knowingly or recklessly inflict bodily injury or serious mental injury.[15] Most laws provide for a temporary restraining

---

*For example, in Tennessee, PTs are required to report suspected cases of abuse under the following statutory mandate: "Any person, including, but not limited to, a physician, nurse, social worker, department personnel, coroner, medical examiner, alternate care facility employee, or caretaker, having reasonable cause to suspect that an adult has suffered abuse, neglect, or exploitation, shall report or cause reports to be made in accordance with the provisions of this part." (Tennessee Code Annotated 71-6-103[b][1].)

†Under Tennessee Code Annotated 71-6-103(b)(1), knowing failure to make a report is a Class A misdemeanor, carrying a penalty of 11 months, 29 days' imprisonment or a fine not to exceed $2,500, or both.

order, which is designed to prevent the abuser from inflicting further injury. Many states provide for protection of the identity of the reporting party.*

In addition to legal intervention, there are a number of things that PTs and administrators can do to combat the problem of elder abuse in their communities. Staff education regarding elder abuse is crucial. Staff should also be educated regarding conflict resolution, dealing with difficult patient situations, and stress management.[16] Screening efforts are also encouraged: the AMA has suggested that all older adults be asked by their physicians about family violence, even if there are no observable symptoms. A number of service-oriented strategies have been directed at reducing elder abuse; PTs are involved in these efforts professionally or on a volunteer basis. Many of the strategies are designed to enable elders to live as independently as possible for as long as possible, including (1) aging resource centers, (2) adult day-care centers, (3) home delivered meals, (4) chore services, (5) home care, (6) neighborhood visiting teams, (7) calling teams, (8) roommate matching services, and (9) fall risk screening and intervention. Once care is required, other supports may be needed, such as respite care and support groups for caregivers. Also helpful are special law enforcement and multidisciplinary hospital-based abuse teams skilled in dealing with issues of abuse.

Some statutes also address the individual who requests that no report be made. Under Tennessee law, if the adult does not consent to protective services, the service is terminated unless the individual lacks consent and is in imminent danger.[17] This provision leaves the determination to the department of human services and does not relieve the reporter of the duty to report the suspected abuse.

Legal capacity to consent to services requires a case-by-case factual determination. This may be a difficult matter to determine, as illustrated by a case involving an elderly woman suffering from gangrene of the feet.[18] Her physicians recommended amputation, for which she refused to give consent, and a trial court granted permission for the surgery. The appellate court justices interviewed the woman, Mrs. Northern, during her appeal and determined that she was generally lucid and of sound mind and that she expressed a strong desire to live. However, as to the matter of her feet, "her comprehension is blocked, blinded, or dimmed to the extent that she is incapable of recognizing facts which would be obvious to a person of normal perception."[18] The court did not authorize the surgery but rather appointed a person to

---

*See, for example, Tennessee Code Annotated 71-6-118, stating that the identity of a party reporting abuse shall remain confidential unless a court so orders for good cause shown.

act on Mrs. Northern's behalf if the condition became so critical as to demand immediate amputation to save her life.

Application to Case 4.1

If Elaine lives in a state with a mandatory reporting law that applies to PTs, she must report the suspected abuse to the appropriate state authorities. (Some states permit hospital employees to report abuse to their supervisors, as long as a hospital representative then makes the required report.) As noted, many states keep the identity of the reporter confidential. Many offer civil and criminal immunity to the reporter, if the report is made in good faith.*

The case of Frieda Simms poses a potential ethical dilemma for Elaine. She may be required by law to report suspected abuse, yet she may be aware that her community lacks the resources to provide her elderly patient with a viable alternative caretaker. Furthermore, she may suspect that the abuser will intensify his abuse if he learns of the investigation; she may even fear for her own safety. Failure to report may result in a fine or imprisonment, or both; many states make failure to report suspected abuse under a mandatory reporting law a misdemeanor.

ETHICAL ANALYSIS

In resolving her ethical dilemma, Elaine might employ the six-step process outlined in the first chapter. Suppose that Frieda has asked Elaine not to disclose the abuse to anyone. In the first step of this process, Elaine must determine if this is primarily an ethical problem. There is little doubt that this poses an ethical problem; clearly the dilemma concerns right or wrong behavior. However, it is worth noting that Elaine may conceive of the dilemma as whether to pursue her own self-interest (for example, not to get involved) or whether to pursue moral action. In that case, the dilemma might be more like a hard choice.

The second step of the process involves the generation of options. From the systems perspective, there are three major models for dealing with the problem of elder abuse: the spousal-abuse model, the advocacy model, and the adult-protection model.[12] The spousal-abuse model involves removing the victim from the home. In the advocacy model, a neutral counselor explains the victim's rights and assists in

---

*See, for example, Alabama Code 38-9-9.

finding appropriate community resources. Mandatory reporting represents the adult-protection model. Elaine's major options are to

1. Report the violence to the appropriate agency (adult-protection model).
2. Discuss the options with Frieda, referring her as appropriate to other agencies, or honor her request to keep the information in confidence (advocacy model).
3. Have Frieda removed from the abusive situation (spousal-abuse model).

The third step calls for the identification of major duties, rights, consequences, and virtues. The duties and options can be described in terms of beneficence, nonmaleficence, and autonomy. A part of the obligation to autonomy is the duty to maintain confidentiality—that is, a part of self-determination is the right to determine whether personal information should be shared with others. Accordingly, the American Physical Therapy Association's (APTA) *Guide for Professional Conduct*[19] deals with confidential information as a part of Principle 1 (1.2A, C, and D), which relates to respect for the rights and dignity of individuals: "Information relating to the PT-patient relationship is confidential and may not be communicated to a third party not involved in that patient's care without the prior written consent of the patient, subject to applicable law" (1A). Section 1.2C of the same section states that "[i]nformation derived from the working relationships of PTs shall be held confidential by all parties." However, the final section (1.2D) delineates certain exceptions to the duty of confidentiality: "Information may be disclosed to appropriate authorities when it is necessary to protect the welfare of an individual or the community. Such disclosure shall be in accordance with applicable law."[19]

If Elaine breaks Frieda's confidence and reports the abuse (adult-protection model), or has Frieda removed from her home (spousal-abuse model), the possible consequences are

1. Loss of trust on an individual and societal level. Frieda's trust in Elaine will be seriously eroded. One of the historical arguments for confidentiality is the consequentialist argument that confidentiality ensures that patients can safely seek medical advice and reveal information pertinent to their care.[20]
2. Frieda may experience increased violence and retaliation (a common occurrence in domestic violence).
3. Frieda may lose her home, be institutionalized, or suffer other negative changes in lifestyle.
4. Frieda may avoid future health care, causing adverse effects to her health.

The adult-protection and spousal abuse models represent forms of paternalism, seriously undermining Frieda's autonomy (many elder abuse laws are modeled after or are part of child abuse laws). The assumption that elders are necessarily incompetent is a type of ageism.[11]

If Elaine were to decide on option 2 (advocacy model), some of the possible consequences of her action are

1. Frieda may decide not to pursue help, which may lead to physical harm.
2. If the law requires Elaine to report through legal channels, she may be in violation of the law.

The advocacy model preserves autonomy at the possible expense of beneficence and nonmaleficence.

In the fourth step of the process, conflicts are identified. In this case, the conflicts are between preserving autonomy by maintaining confidentiality and nonmaleficence in preventing physical harm to Frieda. Additional conflicts are between the obligation to obey the law (a kind of societal beneficence) and beneficence on the individual level.

The final two steps of the process involve moral ingenuity and final selection of a course of action. One option is to discuss services available in the community or to set up a discussion involving a social worker, minister, or counselor. If the daughter is also a victim of abuse, a referral can be made to the local domestic violence shelter or a work retraining program. A social worker may be helpful to the client and to the PT in identifying community resources.

Several guidelines may be used in the process of selecting a course of action. As Beauchamp and Childress[21] pointed out, a part of this process is weighing the probability of and magnitude of harm. As the probability and magnitude of harm increase, so also the duty to breach confidentiality increases. Examples of significant probability and magnitude of harm frequently involve patients under psychiatric care who have threatened violence against a specifically identified individual.[22] In this case, determination of probability and magnitude of harm should include a consideration of whether the victim is competent, the cognitive ability of the patient, the type and severity of abuse, and the frequency of abuse.[12]

With regard to elder abuse, several facts are pertinent. A report from the General Accounting Office indicates that mandatory reporting laws are less effective in decreasing elder abuse than education programs aimed at both patients and providers.[11] The implication for this case is that breaking Frieda's confidentiality for the goal of protecting her from harm may not be effective. Accordingly, Elaine may be in a situation in which the most ethical option is not legal in her state.

QUESTIONS FOR FURTHER REFLECTION

1. How should Elaine determine whether Frieda is at significant risk for injury? How should Elaine measure the probability and magnitude of harm to Frieda?

2. What resources are available in your community to assist victims and perpetrators of child abuse, wife abuse, and elder abuse?

3. Have you experienced situations in which you felt obligated to breach confidentiality?

4. In this situation, what steps should precede Elaine's breaching confidentiality?

5. In response to the increasing violence in society, the AMA has promoted physician screening for domestic violence. Do PTs have a responsibility to screen for elder abuse or other kinds of domestic violence?

6. What questions would you ask to screen for domestic violence? For elder abuse? For child abuse?

7. What is the law in your state regarding abuse reporting? What are your facility's policies regarding suspected abuse?

EMPLOYMENT ISSUES

The previous section addressed the abuse of power as domestic violence. In domestic violence, a spouse, family member, or significant other abuses power in the personal sphere. Employers may also exercise power over employees in inappropriate ways. Frequently, this abuse of power is directed against minority groups or women, who historically have been the victims of oppression. Many employment practices and laws attempt to prevent this type of abuse of power, either conscious or unconscious, in the work setting. This section addresses employment issues, such as hiring and firing, which present the opportunity to wield power.

Employment Law

Employment issues are a critical matter for administrators. Employment law is a complex area, involving federal constitutional law and civil rights statutes, supplemented by regulations and cases of the National Labor Relations Board, judicial cases, as well as state constitutional provisions and civil rights statutes.

Administrators frequently ask, "How do I fire an unacceptable employee?" Somewhat paradoxically, the best time to begin documentation to support firing an employee is before he or she is hired. The employer should be able to show, during all phases of employment, that individuals are treated equally and without regard to impermissible classifications. Workers must be shown to meet the bona fide occupational qualifications of the position.[23]

Hiring, Performance Review, and Firing

Without a written employment contract, most employment relationships fall under the employment-at-will theory.* The rule is that when an employment relationship is not defined by a fixed duration or an agreed limit on the right of either party to terminate it, the relationship can be terminated at will by either party, at any time, for any reason. However, discrimination statutes prohibit termination on the basis of race, national origin, gender, pregnancy, religion, age, disability, and marital status. These statutes include Title VII of the Civil Rights Act of 1964,[24] the Age Discrimination in Employment Act,[25] the Rehabilitation Act of 1973,[26] and the Americans with Disabilities Act (ADA).†[27] Additionally, case law prohibits termination for reasons that violate public policy, such as interference with workers' compensation and other statutory rights or for reporting Occupational Safety and Health Administration (OSHA) violations.

Employment applications and interviews should be designed to determine the applicant's specific qualifications for the job. Ask yourself whether the information pertains to a job-related characteristic. Avoid questions regarding attributes protected by discrimination laws, including race, religion, gender, pregnancy, and date of birth. Do not require that a photograph be submitted with an application. It is acceptable to ask about an individual's authorization to work in the United States but not about national origin or citizenship status. The ADA and its precursor, the Rehabilitation Act of 1973, prohibit inquiries regard-

---

*Note that promises made in employee handbooks have been construed as contractual obligations.

†Employers are also subject to other employment laws that are beyond the scope of this book, including the Family and Medical Leave Act, the Occupational Safety and Health Act, the Fair Labor Standards Act, and the Labor-Management Relations Act.

ing an applicant's disability status, injury record, or worker's compensation claims filed.

In a 1995 Texas case, a jury awarded a plaintiff $45,000 in damages after a prospective employer asked inappropriate interview questions.[28] The plaintiff, Timothy Burke, applied for a position as a retail sales representative with the Community Coffee Company. Mr. Burke had facial weakness, visual and hearing impairments, and paralysis secondary to removal of a brain tumor years before his application. Company representatives told Mr. Burke they were uncomfortable with his appearance and asked him to describe how it happened and the treatment he received. They also reportedly asked other insensitive questions regarding the condition. Mr. Burke did not receive a job offer; however, the jury did not find that the company violated the ADA by not hiring Mr. Burke, only that company representatives had made unlawful pre-employment inquiries.

After an individual is hired, performance evaluations should provide an employee with notice of unsatisfactory performance and with an opportunity for the employee to improve. To provide effective documentation for an employer in litigation, evaluations must show that employees were treated consistently. The review process should be thorough and objective, based on specific job performance criteria. Supervisors should be trained to make effective evaluations. Employees should be asked to sign all reviews and to document comments on the review form. Decisions regarding promotions must also pass muster under the ADA and other civil rights statutes.

When an individual leaves an employer, supervisors may be asked to respond to requests for reference. The safest policy is to provide only dates of employment and job title. Any additional information offered should be verified for accuracy and released only to individuals with a legitimate, business-related need to know. The former employee should provide written authorization for release of the information. If the reference information is given over the telephone, the caller's identity should be verified.

CASE FOR FURTHER REFLECTION

Tara Sawyer is the director of a physical therapy department in an acute care hospital. The department consists of four PTs, two PTAs, and the director, all women in their twenties and thirties. Tara has been authorized to hire one additional PT to fill a recent vacancy. She has learned that the hospital is planning to institute a hiring freeze, so Tara is particularly concerned that she hire just the right person to fit well within the department.

In creating a classified advertisement to fill the position, what criteria should be used to select candidates for interview?

What interview questions are allowed? What interview questions should be avoided?

Persons with Disabilities

CASE 4.2

Lisa Lauro is a PT and a wound specialist. During wound debridement, she cut herself with the scalpel. The patient was seropositive for human immunodeficiency virus (HIV), and Lisa subsequently tested positive. Lisa's supervisor removed her from wound care duties and offered her an alternate position with the same salary and benefits. Lisa declined, asserting that the risk of transmission of HIV is extremely small and noting that she had spent considerable time and effort to develop a specialized expertise. What are the legal and ethical issues raised?

The Rehabilitation Act of 1973 provides that no otherwise qualified handicapped individual may be denied benefits or be subject to discrimination by reason of the handicap under any program receiving funds from the federal government.[26] The act is thus applicable to most hospitals and universities. A handicapped individual is defined as one who has a physical or mental impairment that substantially limits one or more of the major life activities or has a record of such an impairment or is regarded as having a handicap.[29]

The ADA was enacted in 1990 to expand opportunities for individuals with disabilities in the areas of employment, public accommodation, transportation, access to state and local services, and telecommunications.[30] The employment provisions of the ADA (Title I) apply to all employers with 15 or more employees.*

The ADA defines disability as a physical or mental impairment that substantially limits one or more major life activities, a record of such impairment, or being regarded as having a disability.[31] Disability includes emotional or mental illness and specific learning disabilities, a history of such disabilities, or a history of alcohol or drug use. People using drugs illegally, however, are not protected under the ADA, and use of alcohol at the workplace is specifically prohibited.[32] Thus, the second circuit court of appeals upheld a hospital's firing of an alcoholic physician who had been intoxicated at the hospital.[33]

---

*Title II relates to provision of state and local services and is not covered specifically in this book. (Note, however, that state or municipal hospitals are required to comply with this section.) Title III, discussed in Chapter 6, relates to places of public accommodation.

The ADA requires employers to make reasonable modifications, as needed, to their policies, practices, and procedures to accommodate persons with disabilities.[34] These might include auxiliary aides for communication or removal of architectural barriers. However, facilities need not fundamentally alter the nature of the services provided. Modifications must be achievable without undue hardship—that is, significant difficulty or expense.[35] Factors to be considered include the nature and cost of the proposed modifications, the overall financial resources of the company, the type of operation, and the impact.

In *Reigel v. Kaiser Foundation Health Plan of North Carolina*[36] the court found that a physician's former employer, a medical group, need not restrict her duties to supervision or provide a full-time assistant to accommodate her disability. (The physician was an internist suffering from reflex sympathetic dystrophy of the right arm.) The court expressly noted that the ADA does not require involuntary restructuring or hiring two persons to do tasks ordinarily assigned to one person.

Between the inception of the ADA and early 1995, the Equal Employment Opportunity Commission (EEOC) received almost 30,000 complaints of employment discrimination under the act.[37] Thirty-four percent had a finding of no cause, 26 cases were in court, and 200 more were expected to go to trial. During this period, the U.S. Justice Department had received 2,400 complaints under the public service accommodations provisions, most of which were settled through voluntary compliance.[37]

What do typical accommodations cost? A 1994 study based on the experience of Sears, Roebuck showed that the average ADA accommodation cost the company $121; 69% of accommodations cost nothing, 27% cost less than $1,000, and 3% exceeded $1,000.[38] Table 4.1 illustrates the most commonly cited ADA violations and impairments.

In 1995, a Michigan court determined that a hospital was justified in discharging an HIV-positive operating room surgical technician.*[39] The technician had refused an alternative accommodating position at a similar salary. The hospital released the technician due to the real possibility of transmission, the severity of his illness, and the fact that the disability was related to his ability to perform the job. The court found that the hospital's actions did not violate the ADA, the Rehabilitation Act, or Michigan law.

---

*See also *Bradley v. University of Tex. M.D. Anderson Cancer Ctr.*, 3 F.3d 922 (5th Cir.) (1993), [cert. denied], 114 S.Ct. 1071 (U.S. 1994).

Table 4.1
Cumulative Americans with Disabilities Act (ADA) charge data as
of December 31, 1994

	Number	*Percent of Total**
ADA Violations Most Often Cited		
Discharge	20,171	50.5
Failure to provide reasonable accommodation	10,264	25.7
Hiring	4,364	10.9
Harassment	4,294	10.8
Discipline	2,947	7.4
Layoff	2,069	5.2
Benefits	1,576	3.9
Promotion	1,495	3.7
Rehire	1,472	3.7
Wages	1,385	3.5
Suspension	910	2.3
Impairments Most Often Cited		
Back	7,799	19.5
Neurologic	4,824	12.1
Emotional and psychiatric	4,569	11.4
Extremities	2,934	7.3
Heart	1,833	4.6
Diabetes	1,437	3.6
Substance abuse	1,416	3.6
Hearing	1,231	3.1
Vision	1,148	2.9
Blood disorders	1,054	2.6
HIV (subcategory of blood disorder)	729	1.8
Cancer	970	2.4
Asthma	714	1.8

*Percents do not total 100 because individuals can allege multiple violations and
because the list of impairments is incomplete.
HIV = human immunodeficiency virus.

Application to Case 4.2

It is possible that a court considering Lisa's potential claims under the
Rehabilitation Act or the ADA would determine that no violation has
occurred if the hospital chooses to terminate her employment after
offering an acceptable alternative. Invasive work is an intrinsic part of
her current position and cannot be readily accommodated. ADA cases,
however, are extremely fact specific and thus difficult to generalize.[40]
What constitutes an undue burden for one employer may not for
another. Individual characteristics of the employer will be considered

in a liability determination. The court will also look to Centers for Disease Control (CDC) guidelines in consideration of this matter (see *Ethical Analysis*).

The ethical issue from the standpoint of the director is to balance Lisa's autonomy with nonmaleficence with regard to patients. These principles find their professional basis in the APTA's *Code of Ethics* and *Guide for Professional Conduct* injunctions to respect the dignity of each individual, not to discriminate against others, and to put the welfare of the patient first (1.1B and 1.1C). The APTA House of Delegates issued the following Position on Physical Therapy Practitioners with Communicable Diseases or Conditions (HOD 06-93-15-20) in 1993:

> Physical therapists and physical therapist assistants with known communicable diseases or conditions have a right to continue careers in physical therapy in a capacity which poses no identifiable risk to their patients.
>
> Physical therapists and physical therapist assistants with known communicable diseases or conditions shall have an ethical obligation to abstain from those professional activities over which they cannot sustain an acceptable level of risk of transmission to the patient. An acceptable level of risk is achieved by exercising precautions recommended by the Centers for Disease Control and Prevention,* the Occupational Health and Safety Administration, or other authoritative body.
>
> Physical therapists and physical therapist assistants who are both at risk of acquiring communicable diseases or conditions and who engage in professional activities with identifiable risks of transmission of those communicable diseases or conditions should take appropriate measures to determine their health status.

Lisa and her supervisor disagree on the issue of what constitutes an acceptable risk of transmission. However, it should be noted that there is some ambiguity within the position statement itself. One portion of the position suggests that the goal is "acceptable level of risk" as guided by CDC and OSHA requirements. However, the first portion of the position suggests that the acceptable risk is in fact "no identifiable risk to their patients." Lisa and her supervisor may both claim a basis in the position.

---

*CDC guidelines mandate that HIV-positive health care workers who engage in exposure-prone procedures should seek counsel from an expert review panel before continuing such procedures. Prospective patients would have to be notified of the health care worker's seropositive status. "In practice, this negates their ability to do any exposure prone procedure."[41] An exposure-prone procedure is one that is likely to expose a patient to a health care worker's blood; for example, invasive procedures lasting longer than 2.5–3.0 hours, especially when blood loss exceeds 250–300 ml, or that involve the simultaneous presence of a sharp instrument in a poorly visualized or confined anatomic site.

QUESTIONS FOR FURTHER REFLECTION

1. What resources might Lisa and her supervisor use to determine the real risk to patients in Lisa's job?

2. What is the difference between acceptable risk and no identifiable risk to patients? Which of these standards should guide decisions?

3. How might this dilemma be resolved?

4. What are Lisa's responsibilities to the patient? How can Lisa avoid being guided by her self-interest alone?

5. How can the supervisor avoid being guided by irrational fears?

CASE 4.3

Linda Frame is the director of physical therapy for a large extended care facility. She is employed by a national rehabilitation corporation that is seeking a new regional director of rehabilitation services. Linda's supervisor, Bill Wharton, suggests to her that the job could be hers in exchange for sexual favors. He also indicates that the company has considered eliminating the director position Linda currently occupies and that she may lose her job if she is not selected for the promotion. What legal remedies does Linda have available to her?

LEGAL ANALYSIS: SEXUAL HARASSMENT

Definition and Incidence

Under federal law, unwelcome sexual advances, sexual favors, or other verbal or physical conduct of a sexual nature constitute harassment when

1. Submission is an implied or overt requirement to continued employment or advancement (quid pro quo), *or*
2. It has the purpose or effect of unreasonably interfering with work performance or creating an intimidating, hostile, or offensive working environment (hostile workplace).

Prevalence data vary; however, most reports indicate that sexual harassment is a serious issue for employers. A study from the *American*

Journal of Psychiatry found that 42% of women and 15% of men were affected by occupational sexual harassment, blue collar and white collar workers alike.[42] In a national study of PTs by deMayo, 63% of PTs surveyed had experienced at least one incident of sexual harassment.[43] A study of physicians reported that 73% of women and 22% of men suffered from harassment during medical training; only 1–7% of victims filed complaints.[42] The effects of sexual harassment may be serious; in addition to employment difficulties, one study suggested that such harassment produces psychological and physical symptoms in 90% of its victims.[44]

Determining just what constitutes sexual harassment may be difficult, particularly in the case of a hostile workplace environment. The U.S. Supreme Court considered the matter in a 1993 case arising at a forklift company in Nashville.[45] The company president told a female employee, "You're a woman; what do you know?" called her a "dumbass woman," and suggested that they go to the Holiday Inn to negotiate her raise. He routinely asked female employees to get change out of his front pants pocket for him and dropped objects on the floor and asked female employees to pick them up while he watched. In determining whether this constituted a hostile workplace, the Supreme Court ruled that the plaintiff need not show psychological harm or injury to prevail. Rather, the presence or absence of psychological harm or injury is considered as one factor among several, including frequency and severity of harassment, whether the conduct is physically threatening or humiliating (or merely offensive), and whether it interferes with work performance.

In determining whether conduct is reasonable, whose standard is applied, a man's or a woman's? At least two circuit courts have ruled that the reasonableness of conduct should be judged by what a reasonable woman would consider harassment (assuming a woman is the victim).[46, 47] These courts considered that women's perceptions of sexual contact occur against a backdrop of coercion and sexual assault, making women particularly vulnerable regarding sexual advances that occur in workplace.[47] Recognizing that some sexually harassing conduct may not be intentional, these courts nonetheless look to the victim's perspective. However, this issue has not yet been decided by the Supreme Court, and the circuit courts are split. Note that in *Harris*, the Supreme Court referred to a reasonable person's standard without specifically addressing the issue. The Supreme Court has agreed to review a ruling by the Fifth Circuit Court of Appeals that sexual harassment by a supervisor of the same gender does not constitute sexual harassment under Title VII.[48]

Employer Duties

What is an employer to do? Employers have a duty to express strong disapproval of sexual harassment and to develop appropriate policies and sanctions. Employers may be liable for failing to remedy or prevent a hostile work environment that management knew of or should have known about, in the exercise of reasonable care.[49]

Employers must fully investigate complaints, issue written warnings to refrain, and reprimand as appropriate (e.g., through suspension or probation). The regulations do not require immediate firing of harassers; however, telling the harasser to stay away from the person being harassed without following up is considered insufficient.

Application to Case 4.3

Case 4.3 appears to constitute quid pro quo sexual harassment. Linda is being asked to submit to sexual advances in exchange for a promotion and, perhaps, to retain her current position. If the employer had knowledge of Bill Wharton's behavior, the company is at risk as well. If the employer is found to have engaged in employment discrimination, the employer is liable for lost earnings and other benefits. The employer may be ordered to reinstate or promote an aggrieved individual. If the discrimination is considered intentional, compensatory and punitive damages may also be available.

ETHICAL ANALYSIS

Case 4.3 involves the problems of gender in society, where men have historically exercised power over women. It represents a case of injustice and infringement of autonomy and dignity through the abuse of power in the workplace. At one time, Linda would have had no legal recourse. Although few people would say that Linda would be wrong to take legal action against her boss and the company, it is true that litigation might hurt Linda's future career. The more difficult underlying question is how to bring about changes in society at large and in specific organizational cultures that do not promote justice.

Although a significant number of women are the victims of overt sexual harassment, many more are victims of more subtle forms of sexual discrimination. Women experience difficulty gaining promotion even in traditionally female professions such as social work[50] and physical therapy. White-male–dominated organizational cultures also pose challenges to justice in the workplace. Although the organizational culture may dictate that important decisions are discussed over racquetball and golf, these opportunities may not be open to women, African-Americans, or other minorities; or they may be allowed to participate in these activities without gaining the same benefits from participation.

Experience suggests that the informal structures of organizational cultures change slowly and with difficulty. In addition, many organizations struggle with the collective nature of organizational values. Who is responsible for the direction of institutional decisions, and how is the organizational ethos shaped? Laws and ethical standards are strained in their application to these elements of life.

CASE 4.4

Tom Kerman is a PT who works in an outpatient clinic. He is treating Brenda Caldwell for cervical injuries that she sustained in a work-related accident. Tom and Brenda have started a dating relationship and have become intimate. What legal and ethical problems does this situation pose?

LEGAL ANALYSIS: SEXUAL MISCONDUCT

Definition and Incidence

Sexual misconduct is defined for the purposes of this book as contact of a sexual nature between health care professionals and patients, and sometimes former patients, in which the therapist is motivated by a desire for sexual gratification. The Model Practice Act for Physical Therapy[51] defines sexual misconduct as grounds for disciplinary action and states:

> Engaging in sexual misconduct. Sexual misconduct, for the purpose of this section, includes the following:
>
> 1. Engaging in or soliciting sexual relationships, whether consensual or non-consensual, while a physical therapist or physical therapist assistant/patient relationship exists.
> 2. Making sexual advances, requesting sexual favors, and engaging in other verbal conduct or physical contact of a sexual nature with patients, clients or co-workers.
> 3. Intentionally viewing a completely or partially disrobed patient in the course of treatment if the viewing is not related to patient diagnosis or treatment under current practice standards.

Sexual misconduct is an issue with serious legal and ethical implications that has received relatively little attention in the physical therapy literature. The psychological theory underlying patient attraction to health care professionals is that of transference—that is, the unconscious transfer of emotions regarding significant others to the therapist. While this phenomenon is usually associated with psychotherapy, it does occur in physical therapy.[52]

Why do society and the physical therapy profession want to prohibit relationships of a sexual nature between therapists and their patients? A number of reasons have been suggested in the medical literature. First, the therapist may consciously or unconsciously use the power imbalance inherent in the relationship to influence or coerce the patient into the relationship. The relationship may also interfere with the therapist's clinical judgment regarding that patient. For example, a clinician may fail to refer the patient for a needed consult for fear that the relationship will be discovered. Another reason is that such relationships may diminish the image of health professionals in the eyes of the public—lessening trust. Most important is the issue of harm to the patient. Patients who have been victimized by sexual misconduct often experience feelings of guilt, shame, anger, rage, grief, depression, loss of self-esteem, confusion, fear, and generalized distrust.[44]

Several rather unique aspects of the physical therapy environment may make patients particularly vulnerable. In some settings, PTs may develop close therapeutic relationships with their patients over time. Some patients have cognitive deficits, such as those associated with traumatic brain injury, that impair their judgment about entering such a relationship. Finally, there is the issue of touch; it is used daily in manners therapeutic, encouraging, or congratulatory. Touch is a necessary part of physical therapy practice, but it may send mixed messages to patients and their family members.[53]

Legal Intervention

In examining legal consequences of sexual misconduct, the ways in which states have used criminal law to prohibit sexual misconduct are considered first. Traditional rape and sexual assault charges can be brought against practitioners who engage in nonconsensual sexual activity. For example, a Washington PT was charged with rape for digital penetration of a patient (J. Gillie. "Physical therapist charged with molestation." *The News Tribune* April 1, 1994). Some states have expressly criminalized sexual activity (including consensual activity) between certain health care professionals and their patients; some of these laws apply to physicians only, others to psychotherapists, others to a broader class of health professionals.

Licensure actions are another means for states to discipline therapists for sexual misconduct. At least one state physical therapy practice act specifically prohibits engaging in a sexual act with a patient.*[54] More typically, however, states use generic language in their practice acts, such as "unprofessional conduct," or "conduct involving moral turpitude," to impose licensure restrictions for sexual misconduct. In Tennessee, grounds for disciplinary action of PTs include "unprofessional, dishonorable or unethical conduct," which could be applied in a sexual misconduct case.[55]

State licensure boards may impose discipline despite the absence of clear proof of sexual misconduct. In a case involving a North Carolina dentist, a 90-day suspension was imposed following a complaint that he had administered nitrous oxide to a female patient, indecently exposed himself, and assaulted her.[56] Although the allegations of sexual misconduct were not sufficiently proved, the examiners imposed the sanction on the basis that it was outside the standard of care and, therefore, negligent for the dentist to administer nitrous oxide sedation to a female patient without an acceptable chaperone.

Patients can file civil suits under a variety of legal theories, including battery (nonconsensual touching), sexual assault, malpractice, intentional infliction of emotional distress, and even contract theory in some situations.[57] Some states have adopted a specific civil cause of action for sexual contact with patients, most commonly in psychotherapy or counseling settings. In both criminal and civil statutes addressing sexual misconduct, sexual contact is often not clearly defined.

Application to Case 4.4

Assuming the relationship described in Case 4.4 is consensual, it appears that it would not violate the law in most states. As noted, some state statutes specifically prohibit even consensual sexual relationships between PTs and their patients. Additionally, some state licensure boards may bring a licensure action on the grounds that Tom has engaged in "unprofessional conduct." Of course, the danger to Tom, from a legal risk-management perspective, is that Brenda may later characterize the relationship as something other than consensual, perhaps due to the power imbalance of their professional relationship. She may then seek redress through a variety of civil actions, depending on their availability under state law. These include battery, sexual assault, malpractice, and intentional infliction of emotional distress.

---

*Under Colorado law, grounds for disciplinary action of a PT include engaging in a sexual act with a patient while a patient-PT relationship exists. For this discussion, "patient-PT relationship" means the period of time beginning with the initial evaluation through the termination of treatment. For the purposes of this paragraph, "sexual act" means sexual contact, sexual intrusion, or sexual penetration as defined in section 18-3-401 of Colorado revised statute 12-41-115(1)(b)C.R.S.

ETHICAL ANALYSIS

The *Guide for Professional Conduct*[19] addresses the issue of relationships with patients in section 1.3: "PTs shall not engage in any sexual relationship or activity, whether consensual or nonconsensual, with any patient while a physical therapist-patient relationship exists." Implicitly, the *Guide* acknowledges the power that any provider holds over a patient. This imbalance of power means that no relationship can be truly consensual as long as a therapist/patient relationship exists. The argument is that the power of the professional role undercuts the patient's autonomy and ability to give consent to the relationship. Some state statutes expressly state that a patient is presumed to be unable to provide consent to sexual relations with a health care provider. For example, Florida law provides for discipline of physicians for engaging a patient in sexual activity and states, "A patient shall be presumed to be incapable of giving free, full, and informed consent to sexual activity with his physician."[58]

Writing from the perspective of sexual relationships between obstetricians-gynecologists and patients, McCullough et al.[59] described the challenges to voluntariness in such relationships:

> Voluntariness, in turn, requires that the patient's decision-making process be free of controlling internal psychologic and physical factors and of external factors. Obviously, phenomena such as fear of rejection, vulnerability that understandably could lead a patient to conclude that there was no other alternative, and transference can combine to undermine the voluntariness.... The effect of such internal, psychologic phenomena can be reinforced by the external phenomenon of the physician as an authority figure, whose suggestions, requests, or demands may be very difficult, if not impossible, for the patient to resist.

McCullough et al. noted that the prohibition against sexual relationships between physician and patient rests on both autonomy and beneficence. They rejected this principles-based approach to the problem. Arguing from a virtue-based approach (self-effacement, self-sacrifice, compassion, and integrity on the part of the physician) the authors concluded that physicians have an obligation to put aside feelings of sexual attraction. However, physicians are free to have a sexual relationship with a patient after the professional relationship has been terminated.[59]

Some people believe that it is not appropriate for a health care professional to have a sexual relationship with a patient even after the professional relationship has ended, particularly when the patient is known to be vulnerable (e.g., the victim of prior sexual abuse or with known impairments). This could suggest that, from an ethical standpoint, the real issue may be the nature of the relationship and appropriate boundaries between the therapist and the provider. Gabbard and Nadelson[60] described boundaries and their importance in the following manner:

> Professional boundaries in medical practice are not well defined. In general, they are the parameters that describe the limits of a fiduciary relationship in which one person (a patient) entrusts his or her welfare to another [a provider], to whom a fee is paid for the provision of a service. Boundaries imply professional distance and respect, which, of course, includes refraining from sexual involvement with patients. While sexual contact is perhaps the most extreme form of boundary violation, many other [provider] behaviors may exploit the dependency of the patient on the [provider] and the inherent power differential. These include dual relationships, business transactions, certain gifts and services, some forms of language use, some types of physical contact, time and duration of appointments, location of appointments, mishandling of fees, and misuses of the physical examination.

Another ethical challenge in this area is the problem of correctly identifying how intentions are perceived by the patient. Sexual harassment takes place when the patient perceives that the intention in touching is not therapeutic but sexual in nature. The crux of the matter is not the intention of the provider but the *perception of intention*. Both perception and intention are subjective. The patient's view is given priority because of the power exercised in the relationship by the provider. Therefore, the provider must take every precaution to avoid the possibility of any misperception of intention regarding touch.

QUESTIONS AND NOTES FOR FURTHER REFLECTION

1. Does the *Guide for Professional Conduct* go far enough in prohibiting relationships only with patients currently under treatment?

2. What are the ethical implications of transferring care of a patient to another therapist to date that patient? How would it appear to other patients?

3. Does the patient's diagnosis and length of treatment affect your opinion as to whether it is ethical to have a sexual relationship with a patient? For example, contrast the relationship of Tom and Brenda if Brenda had sustained a C4 quadriplegia and had been under Tom's care for 4 months in a rehabilitation center.

4. What measures should PTs and PTAs take to ensure that patients correctly interpret the nature and intention of their touch?

5. Compare the principle-based approach to sexual relationships between providers and patients to the virtue-based approach

advanced by McCullough et al. What are the relative merits of each approach? Which approach is more compelling to you?

6. Sexual exploitation of patients is frequently preceded by progressive boundary violations of a nonsexual nature, described by Gabbard and Nadelson as a "slippery slope."[60] The same authors noted that attention to nonsexual boundaries may help to avert sexual boundary transgressions. What are specific examples of nonsexual boundary violations in physical therapy?

RISK MANAGEMENT

Risk management refers to those measures taken by institutions and administrators to prevent injuries and to prevent financial loss to the institution.[61] Within the health care setting, an interdisciplinary approach is recommended. One author identified the elements of a risk management program (at the institutional level) as risk control, risk financing, and other administrative functions.[62]

Risk Control

Risk control functions include

- Developing and maintaining an incident report system and other methods of risk identification
- Investigating and analyzing information generated by risk identification systems and recommending necessary corrective action
- Providing advice and assistance to staff on matters involving potential liability
- Reviewing hospital policies and contracts for potential exposure
- Educating staff about risk prevention

Risk Financing

Risk financing functions involve

- Directing and coordinating a hospital's insurance programs
- Directing and monitoring the handling and defense of claims against the hospital
- Analyzing and making recommendations to the administration and board regarding the hospital's risk financing options
- Coordinating the functions of hospital brokers, consultants, and attorneys

Administrative Functions

Administrative functions entail

- Directing and supervising the operations of the risk management department
- Developing and implementing automated systems for tracking risk management data
- Monitoring compliance with regulatory and Joint Commission on Accreditation of Hospitals requirements

Risk Management Strategies

At the departmental level, risk management strategies include[63, 64]

- Early intervention and sympathetic care after accidental injury to a patient
- Preparation of incident reports
- Prompt identification and investigation of specific incidents
- Management of a risk database to identify trends, frequency, and severity
- Formulation and implementation of corrective actions
- Training and educating employees regarding legal duties to patients to assist in reducing exposure
- Maintaining a suggestion box
- Instituting a public relations program
- Developing good interpersonal relationships with patients
- Providing adequate information so that patients understand the course of treatment and expected outcomes
- Making certain that treatment is adequately supervised
- Providing safe premises and equipment
- Keeping good written records

In the case of Tom and Brenda (Case 4.3), what should be done from a risk management perspective to prevent similar cases from occurring? What would you, as a manager, do to ensure that no inappropriate relationships arose in your department and to prevent false accusations of inappropriate sexual conduct?*[65]

To ensure that therapists do not engage in improper relationships with patients and to minimize the risk of false accusations of such relationships, a clear policy that no social or dating relationships with

---

*Note that courts are split regarding the liability of facilities in such cases; recall the notion of respondeat superior; some courts have ruled that employees motivated by professional gratification are not acting within the scope of their employment (see Chapter 2).

patients are permitted should be established. All staff members, including the support staff, should be educated regarding these expectations. The policy should extend to all staff, not just treating therapists. In an Alberta case, a PT with the major ownership interest in a physical therapy clinic was disciplined for a consensual sexual relationship with a patient treated by another therapist.[66]

In formulating risk management approaches, consideration of patient advances is necessary. A 1995 study by deMayo found that 86% of PTs surveyed had experienced some form of inappropriate patient sexual behavior.[43] In a 1993 Canadian study of PTs and PT students, 80.9% of therapists and students reported having encountered some level of inappropriate patient sexual behavior.[67] While nearly half of the therapists and one-third of the students experienced serious inappropriate behaviors (forceful touching, deliberate sexual exposure), only 20% felt harassed. Students were generally less able to recognize harassment than clinicians and also reported more negative effects on work performance as a result. The best strategy to deal with a harasser is to directly confront the harasser, discussing the inappropriateness of the behavior and establishing clear therapeutic boundaries.

Patient modesty and confidentiality must be maintained at all times to avoid even the appearance of improper activity. Some complaints (initiated by family members) may have been prevented by maintenance of professional decorum.

It is crucial to obtain adequate informed consent. Many of the sexual misconduct complaints brought before the judicial committee of the APTA involved myofascial release or sacroiliac mobilization techniques performed near the patient's breast, genitals, or anus.[57] Such procedures should be explained in detail and written informed consent obtained. In another Alberta case, a PT engaged in touching the sternum and pelvis of a female patient while treating her for neck pain. Although no sexual intent was alleged, the therapist was disciplined nonetheless for failing to adequately explain to the patient what he was going to do.[68] Any procedures that involve touching a patient in a manner that could possibly be construed as sexual, even evaluation procedures, must be thoroughly documented.

Whenever possible, patients should be treated by therapists of the same gender. A therapist should listen to his or her "gut feelings" about patients, especially those engaging in excessive inappropriate sexual behavior, and any inappropriate behavior or problem patients should be reported to the supervisor. Scheduling such patients during a busy time of day rather than at the beginning or end of the day, treating them in the clinic rather than bedside, or using chaperones minimizes the risk to both therapist and patient. If all else fails, the patient should be referred to another therapist. In summary, PTs must strive to create and maintain an atmosphere of professional decorum. As PTs, we cannot be afraid to touch, but we must emphasize its healing aspect.

REFERENCES

1. Clark T, Smith McKenna L, Jewell M. Physical therapists' recognition of battered women in clinical settings. Phys Ther 1996;76:12.
2. Tennessee Code Annotated 71-6-102.
3. Tatara T. Understanding the nature and scope of domestic elder abuse with the use of state aggregate data: summaries of state APS and aging agencies. J Elder Abuse Neglect 1993;5:35.
4. Hickey T, Douglass R. In M Kapp (ed), Geriatrics and the Law. New York: Springer, 1992.
5. Pillemer K, Moore D. Abuse of patients in nursing homes: findings from a survey of staff. Gerontologist 1989;29:314.
6. Benton D, Marshall C. Elder abuse. Clin Geriatr Med 1991;7:831.
7. Lachs M, Pillemer K. Abuse and neglect of elderly persons. N Engl J Med 1995;332:437.
8. Elder abuse: abandonment raising public's awareness. Hospitals November 5, 1992;29.
9. AMA Council on Scientific Affairs. Elder abuse and neglect. JAMA 1987; 257:966.
10. Marley MA. Caregiver strain as a predictor of post-hospital functioning of the elderly. D.S.W., diss. Tulane University, 1994.
11. Hyman A, Schillinger D, Lo B. Laws mandating reporting of domestic violence: do they promote patient well-being? JAMA 1995;273:1781.
12. Canadian Task Force on the Periodic Health Examination. Periodic health examination, 1994. Update 4: secondary prevention of elder abuse and mistreatment. Can Med Assoc J 1994;151:1413.
13. 42 U.S.C. 3001 et seq.
14. *Landeros v. Flood*, 551 P.2d 389 (1976).
15. Texas Penal Code 22.04.
16. Silva T. Reporting elder abuse: should it be mandatory or voluntary? Healthspan 1992;9:12.
17. Tennessee Code Annotated 71-6-107.
18. *State Department of Human Services v. Northern*, 563 S.W.2d 197 (Tenn. Ct. App.), [appeal dismissed], 436 U.S. 923, 98 S.Ct. 2816, 56 L.Ed. 2d 767 (1978).
19. American Physical Therapy Association. Guide for Professional Conduct. Alexandria, VA: American Physical Therapy Association, 1997.
20. Kleinman I. Confidentiality and the duty to warn. Can Med Assoc J 1993; 149:1783–1785.
21. Beauchamp TL, Childress JF. Principles of Biomedical Ethics (4th ed). New York: Oxford, 1994;425.
22. *Tarasoff v. Regents of Univ. of Cal.*, 131 Cal.Rptr. 14, 551 P. 2d 334 (1976).
23. Ingram D. Opinions of physical therapy education program directors on essential functions. Phys Ther 1997;77:37.

24. 42 U.S.C.A. §2000e-2000e-7.
25. 29 U.S.C.A. §621-634, 663(a).
26. 29 U.S.C.A. §701-794.
27. 42 U.S.C.A. §12101-12117.
28. *EEOC v. Community Coffee Co., Inc.*, No. H-94 1061 (S.D. Tex. June 28, 1995).
29. Standards for Determining Who Are Handicapped Persons. 28 C.F.R. §41.31(a).
30. Jones D, Watzlaf V, Hobson D, Mazzoni J. Responses within nonfederal hospitals in Pennsylvania to the Americans with Disabilities Act of 1990. Phys Ther 1996;76:49.
31. Nondiscrimination on the Basis of Disability by Public Accommodations in Commercial Facilities—Definitions. 28 C.F.R. §36.104.
32. 42 U.S.C.A. §12114.
33. *Altman v. New York City Health & Hosps. Corp.*, 100 F.3d 1054 (2d Cir. Nov. 21, 1996).
34. Not Making Reasonable Accommodation. 29 C.F.R. §1630.9.
35. Regulations to Implement the Equal Employment Disabilities Act. 29 C.F.R. 1630.2.
36. 859 F. Supp. 963 (E.D.N.C. 1994).
37. National Council on Disability Report. The Americans with Disabilities Act. PT Bull 1995;10.
38. Blanck P. Communicating the Americans with Disabilities Act—transcending compliance: a case report on Sears, Roebuck, and Co. Washington, DC: Annenberg Washington Program, 1994.
39. *Mauro v. Borgess Med. Ctr.*, 886 F. Supp. 1349 (W.D. Mich. 1995).
40. Marone J. Reasonable accommodation in disability law. PT Mag 1995;3:68.
41. Katoma P, Shin Flemmig D. Precautions for the Health Care Worker. In J Fahey, D Shin Flemmig (eds), AIDS/HIV Reference Guide for Medical Professionals (4th ed). Baltimore: Williams & Wilkins, 1997;373.
42. Charney D, Russell R. An overview of sexual harassment. Am J Psychiatry 1994;151:10.
43. deMayo RA. Patient sexual behaviors and sexual harassment: a national survey of physical therapists. Phys Ther 1997;77:739.
44. Pope G. Abuse of psychotherapy: psychotherapist-patient intimacy. Psychother Psychosom 1990;53:191.
45. *Harris v. Forklift Systems, Inc.*, 114 S.Ct. 367 (1993).
46. *Andrews v. City of Philadelphia*, 895 F.2d 1469 (3d Cir. 1990).
47. *Ellison v. Brady*, 924 F.2d 872 (9th Cir. 1991).
48. *Oncale v. Sundowner Offshore Services*, 83 F.3d 118 (5th Cir. 1996).
49. Weddle J. Title VII sexual harassment: recognizing an employer's non-delegable duty to prevent a hostile workplace. Columbia Law Rev 1995;95:724.
50. Thompson JJ, Marley MA. Survival skills for women in human services management. Unpublished paper, 1997.
51. The Federation of State Boards of Physical Therapy. The Model Practice Act for Physical Therapy. Alexandria, VA: The Federation of State Boards of Physical Therapy, 1997.
52. Woltersdorf M. Transference: whistling in the dark. PT Mag 1994;2:61.
53. Knight C. Communicating nonerotic touch to patients. Clin Manage 1989;9(5):20.
54. Colorado Revised Statutes 12-41-115(1)(b)C.R.S.
55. Tennessee Code Annotated 63-13-307(a)(1).

56. *McCollough v. North Carolina State Board of Dental Examiners*, 431 S.E.2d 816 (1993); cert. denied 436 S.E.2d 381 (1993).
57. Scott R. Sexual misconduct. PT Mag 1993;1:78.
58. Florida Statute Annot. 458.331 (j).
59. McCullough LB, Chervenak FA, Coverdale JH. Ethically justified guidelines for defining sexual boundaries between obstetrician-gynecologists and their patients. Am J Obstet Gynecol 1996;175:496.
60. Gabbard GO, Nadelson C. Professional boundaries in the physician-patient relationship. JAMA 1995;273:1445.
61. Risk Management Pearls for Physical Therapists. A Project of the Committee on Risk Management Services and Member Benefits of APTA in Cooperation with the American Society for Healthcare Risk Management. Alexandria, VA: American Physical Therapy Association, 1996;3.
62. Youngberg B. Essentials of Hospital Risk Management. Rockville, MD: Aspen, 1990.
63. Pozgar G. Legal Aspects of Health Care Administration. Gaithersburg, MD: Aspen, 1993.
64. Horsh D. Medico-Legal Aspects of Physical Therapy. In R Hickok (ed), Physical Therapy Administration and Management. Baltimore: Williams & Wilkins, 1974.
65. Schunk C, Propas Parver C. Avoiding allegations of sexual misconduct. Clin Manage 1989;9:19.
66. Decision of the Alberta Discipline Committee. Newsletter May 13, 1995;4.
67. McComas J. Experiences of students and practicing physical therapists with inappropriate patient sexual behavior. Phys Ther 1993;73:762.
68. Decision of the Alberta Discipline Committee. Complaint #92-05. Newsletter July 1993;5.

5

Institutional and Personal Aspects of Patient Rights

This chapter examines a number of issues related to balancing individual rights with societal standards of right and wrong. In addition, the difficulty of ethical decision making when rights and duties conflict is discussed. The first case deals with confidentiality, legal requirements for maintaining privacy of patients' records, and the challenges to both confidentiality and record privacy in a computerized health care environment dominated by managed care. The second case in the chapter explores ethical and legal aspects of death in the case of a patient with terminal lung cancer who has do-not-resuscitate (DNR) orders. In a pluralistic, technologically sophisticated society, death raises difficult ethical and legal questions that have no easy answers. The third case addresses the legal and ethical issues of a burn patient who refuses treatment. In the fourth case, the problem of using restraints with patients who seem to represent a danger to themselves is examined. Discussion focuses on the legal and ethical problems involved in balancing the competing obligations of patient autonomy and protection from injury. Increasingly, hospitals are turning to hospital ethics committees and ethics consultants to provide help in answering questions involving patient rights. This chapter describes the role, composition, process, and limitations of hospital ethics committees and ethics consultation.

CASE 5.1

Larry Dulles is a 26-year-old man being treated in physical therapy for generalized weakness and neurologic problems associated with acquired immunodeficiency syndrome (AIDS). One day his mother took him to therapy. After his treatment session, she remarked to his therapist that he did not seem to be improving. The therapist said, "Well, we don't always see dramatic changes with AIDS patients." Larry's mother was previously unaware of his diagnosis.

What ethical and legal issues are posed by this scenario?

LEGAL ANALYSIS: CONFIDENTIALITY

Legal Intervention

Confidentiality of medical records has traditionally been a matter of state law, with some exceptions, such as drug and alcohol and certain mental health treatment records.* However, the federal Health Insurance Portability and Accountability Act (HIPAA) of 1996 (PL 104-191) required the Department of Health and Human Services (HHS) to issue a report on the matter of medical record confidentiality. The report, issued in October 1997, supported making it a criminal offense, punishable by fines and imprisonment, to disclose individually identifiable health information to another person. The applicability of this provision remains under consideration.

Congressional attention to medical records privacy will be reopened after the HHS report. Congress had previously considered but rejected several proposals to protect medical information. The Medical Records Confidentiality Act, proposed in 1995 by Sen. Robert Bennett of Utah, would have included civil and criminal penalties of up to $10,000 for each violation.[1] Frequent violators could receive fines of up to $250,000 plus exclusion from participation in Medicare and Medicaid.

Some state laws require that all information in a medical record be kept confidential. In addition, many states have express prohibitions on release of certain sensitive information, such as human immunodeficiency virus (HIV) status. Illinois law requires HIV test results to be kept confidential, with certain exceptions, such as in the case of a needle-stick injury of a health care worker. Violation of the confidentiality provision is a Class A misdemeanor.[2] Improper release may also constitute an invasion of privacy or intentional infliction of emotional distress—so-called *intentional torts*. It is particularly important to keep such information private because of ongoing discrimination against individuals suspected of being HIV positive. However, in certain circumscribed instances, the duty to maintain confidentiality can be overridden. In a Texas case, a hospital was not held liable for disclosing the names and addresses of blood donors in a wrongful death action alleging that a patient contracted AIDS from a blood transfusion administered in the hospital.[3]

Violation of state law confidentiality protections may also constitute cause for disciplinary action under the state physical therapy practice act. For example, the District of Columbia Health Professional Licensure Act, which is applicable to physical therapists (PTs), expressly provides for disciplinary action if a licensee willfully breaches a statutory,

---

*Note that certain information regarding alcohol and drug treatment is protected under federal law. See, for example, 42 U.S.C. 290dd-3, 290ee-3.

regulatory, or ethical requirement of confidentiality with respect to a person who is a patient or client of the health professional, unless ordered by the court.[4] The physical therapy practice act in Hawaii provides for discipline for "willfully betraying patient confidentiality."[5] In another jurisdiction, the release of records by a psychologist without her patient's consent was found to violate the state practice act.[6]

Information contained in the medical record is to be kept confidential under ethical norms (see section 1.2 of American Physical Therapy Association's [APTA] *Guide for Professional Conduct*).[7] If it is necessary to impart information to another person, a therapist should seek patient consent and document it. If the patient is unable to give consent, a release must be obtained from a surrogate.

Application to Case 5.1

The therapist's actions in Case 5.1 may violate state laws protecting patient confidentiality, laws specifically protecting information regarding HIV status, or the state physical therapy practice act. In addition, it is likely that the hospital maintains policies regarding patient confidentiality in accord with Joint Commission on Accreditation of Healthcare Organizations (JCAHO) requirements.[8] These violations may subject the therapist to civil fines, criminal penalties, licensure action, and disciplinary action by the hospital. Arguably, Larry could also bring suit under the common law theories of violation of privacy and intentional infliction of emotional distress.

ETHICAL ANALYSIS

Case 5.1 highlights the importance of considering the effects of context and cultural factors on ethical issues. From the discussion of confidentiality in Chapter 4, there can be no doubt that the therapist in this case has violated confidentiality by disclosing information to the mother. This information was divulged casually and without reflection on the issues involved. A major challenge in health care is balancing the need to collaborate (beneficence) with the duty to protect patient confidentiality and privacy (autonomy and nonmaleficence). The therapist's response in Case 5.1 represents collaboration, based in part on her assumptions about the relationship between Larry and his mother.

In the current health care environment, there is an ongoing tension between the obligation to work collaboratively with the patient and family members and the duty to maintain patient confidentiality. As part of the shift from paternalism toward emphasis on patients' rights, health care has increasingly recognized the importance of including the patient in decisions regarding the patient's care. By extension, the importance of considering the family in the context of a functional environment is recognized. Inclusion of the home and family environment is considered critical in planning for discharge from rehabilitation. In evaluating patients, PTs consider what resources the home environment offers, and who will be available to help. Unconsciously, PTs may bring their own experience and assumptions about the role of the family to this process.

Families play different roles in the lives of different cultures and individuals. In some cultures, individuals maintain close contact with a large extended family, but even individuals in those cultures may be estranged or distant from their families. Personal history produces unique dynamics among individual family members. While some siblings share intimate details with each other, others may share very little. Some families have big secrets (e.g., incest) that become the center of dysfunctional relationships within the family. Gay men and lesbians may have particularly complex relationships with family because of potential fear of disapproval of their lifestyle. It is common for some family members to be aware that a patient is gay, while other family members may not know.

The intricacies of relationships and information sharing among families and significant others suggest that PTs need to consider carefully the manner in which they collaborate about rehabilitation issues. Although it is usually possible to balance the demands of collaboration and confidentiality, the right to confidentiality must normally take precedence over collaboration when one is forced to choose between the two. This is particularly important to keep in mind when dealing with patients whose diagnosis carries any kind of perceived or real public stigma. In these cases, it is helpful to give some consideration in advance as to how one can most effectively collaborate and what information can be shared. It may prove helpful to confer with the patient to learn with whom, if anyone, the patient wants the provider to communicate about plans for discharge. As previously noted, this consent-to-share information should be documented.

Although the patient's right to confidentiality is paramount, there are some situations in which considerations of beneficence or nonmaleficence should take precedence. Primarily, these are situations in which society in general or a particular individual is placed at a significant risk of injury by virtue of maintaining patient confidentiality. For example, in the situation of Larry Dulles in Case 5.1, suppose that the therapist had been talking with Larry's wife, Sharon, rather than his mother, and it became clear that Sharon did not realize that Larry has AIDS. Does the therapist or physician have an ethical obligation to disclose the risk of infection to Sharon?

The organizational culture of health care does not always promote patient confidentiality. In an effort to promote teamwork, health care workers may casually discuss patient care issues in public areas. A study of conversations on hospital elevators found that in 259 elevator trips 39 (13.9% of the rides) inappropriate remarks were made.[9] Of these, 18 involved violations of patient confidentiality. The other inappropriate comments raised doubts about other health care providers, were derogatory about the quality of care of the institution, or were derogatory about patients. This is an indication of the way that casual conversation can become a major ethical issue.

The increasing use of computers to maintain medical records creates both opportunities and challenges for medicine. President Bill Clinton's health care reform proposal called for the creation of a national medical database, and many facilities are moving to computer-based patient records (CPRs). Woodward[10] pointed out that the number of people authorized to read the medical record has increased markedly since the 1980s, due in part to increased third party payment for services. The increase in CPRs means that many more people have access to patient medical records. It is difficult to secure computer systems, and in many hospitals literally thousands of health care workers have access to patient information. Woodward pointed out that the interests of society are also served by protecting confidentiality:

> Generally, claims that are meant to protect the individual against the collective weight of society or government are couched in the language of rights. But even if we limit ourselves to the language of interests, a case can and should be made for the interest that society has in protecting privacy. In the medical arena it is easy to rationalize data gathering as an activity undertaken for the sake of the individual and society. But information may be used for many purposes that are not benevolent, and the collection of medical data can easily turn into medical surveillance. Such surveillance, in turn, can lead to unprecedented forms of supervision of personal life.[10]

As Woodward noted, the call for databases to assess outcomes and effectiveness may not be as benign or as beneficial as its billing suggests. These are undoubtedly the types of concerns that have prompted passage of the HIPAA, although it remains unclear as to how this bill will be implemented.

CASE 5.2

Ellen Poole is a 69-year-old woman with terminal lung cancer. She is admitted to the hospital in acute respiratory distress and, once stabilized medically, transferred to the subacute unit. Lillian Dugger is a PT temporarily staffing the subacute unit. She sees Mrs. Poole for progressive ambulation. Lillian is aware that Mrs.

Poole has a living will and a DNR order placed on her chart. During a therapy session, Mrs. Poole becomes unresponsive. Lillian initiates CPR, believing that the DNR order should be disregarded, based on her own religious convictions.

LEGAL ANALYSIS: END-OF-LIFE ISSUES

The public attention to Dr. Kevorkian's "death machine" and the U.S. Supreme Court consideration of physician-assisted euthanasia have rekindled public awareness of the so-called right-to-die cases and reopened questions about medical decision making at the end of life. This area is important for consideration by PTs, not just as an intriguing philosophical and moral issue, but as a practical matter. PTs may be faced with decisions about whether to follow advance directives and may be called on to advise patients concerning advance directives. Questions regarding a patient's rehabilitation potential take on heightened significance when the patient is contemplating execution of an advance directive.

This section describes major right-to-die cases and the Patient Self-Determination Act. The issues of medical futility, liability issues, and physician-assisted suicide are also discussed.

Case Law

The precedent-setting legal case involving the right to die is the case of Karen Ann Quinlan.[11] This young woman had severe brain damage after an overdose of diazepam (Valium) and alcohol, which placed her in a persistive vegetative state. Her father petitioned the court for judicial approval to disconnect his daughter's respirator. The New Jersey Supreme Court permitted him to act as her surrogate decision maker absent a clear written directive, based on a constitutional right of privacy and Karen's right to self-determination; this right includes the right to decline medical treatment. The court noted that the right is not absolute and may be balanced against state interests, including the state's interest in preserving life.

Nancy Cruzan was a 20-year-old woman involved in an automobile accident who was also in a persistent vegetative state.[12] Five years after her injury, Nancy's parents petitioned for removal of artificial nutrition and hydration. The trial court granted permission for the removal, but on appeal the Missouri Supreme Court found that there was not clear and convincing evidence that removal of feeding tubes reflected what

Nancy would have wanted; the decision of the lower court was reversed.[13] (The testimony presented as to Nancy's wishes was that of a former roommate, who said that Nancy had indicated she would not want to live as a "vegetable.")

The case was appealed to the U.S. Supreme Court. The Court found that, if Nancy were competent, her wishes would govern care as patients do have a right to removal of life-sustaining medical treatment, including artificial nutrition and hydration. However, the Court also ruled that states may establish their own evidentiary standard for patient's wishes. In other words, states can require petitioners to show by "clear and convincing" evidence what the comatose individual would have wanted. The Supreme Court thus upheld the Missouri Supreme Court decision.[12]

After the Supreme Court decision, Nancy's parents returned to the lower court presenting additional testimony from Nancy's coworkers to support the request to remove the tube. The court found the evidence to be clear and convincing and the tube was removed. Nancy died 12 days later.

Advance Directives

In 1990, Congress enacted the Patient Self-Determination Act.[14] This statute leaves to the states the right to determine standards for advance directives and withholding of treatment decision making. Furthermore, it requires certain facilities, including hospitals, nursing homes, hospice programs, and home health agencies, to inform patients about applicable state laws governing advance directives. The law also applies to managed care organizations, which must inform new enrollees of the applicable state laws.

What are advance directives? Typically, advance directives refer to living wills and durable powers of attorney for health care. A living will is a document that specifies those medical interventions that individuals would want performed or withheld and the circumstances under which they would want such measures withheld should they become decisionally incapacitated. A durable power of attorney for health care appoints a surrogate decision maker for health care decisions. State laws generally provide for one or the other or both. When such a document exists, it is intended to govern medical decision making as long as it is not shown that it was signed under coercion, or, in the case of a durable power of attorney, that the surrogate is acting in bad faith. Many state laws provide immunity from liability for following advance directives. Although typically defined as documents, ideally advance directives involve a process of communication with the individual's primary physician and others integrally involved in care decisions, including family members.[15]

Of course, difficulties arise when such documents are not present. Variations exist in state law regarding the proof required to establish a patient's wishes without such a document. This can lead to petitions to move a patient to another jurisdiction in which the law is less stringent. Some state laws provide for an individual (typically the spouse or adult child) to make decisions regarding medical care following decisional incapacity even without advance directives. The vast majority of such cases are decided in this manner, between family and physician, and are never presented for judicial determination. Difficulties arise when there are conflicts among family members, when a surrogate appears to be acting in bad faith, or when there is no available surrogate.

There is research suggesting that many advance directives are simply not followed by physicians.[16, 17] Some reasons for such noncompliance with advance directives are that the expressed preference may be too restrictive to allow care that the family or provider believes to be appropriate at the moment of illness, the family or provider does not believe the preferred care would be beneficial, patients or family change their minds, or clinicians are unaware that an advance directive exists (especially with patients transferred from an extended care to an acute care facility).[16–18] Hospital staff may be hesitant to fulfill patients' wishes due to fear of liability, or there may be family disagreement, especially if the written directive is vague.

It is difficult to predict what patients would want based solely on age or medical condition. In one study of nursing home patients, the factors patients considered most important in making treatment decisions were the level of future cognitive functioning and the permanence of the treatment procedure.[19] The nursing home residents surveyed were less inclined to opt for treatment as the projected future level of cognitive functioning declined, and less inclined to opt for permanent tube feeding over temporary tube feeding.[19, 20]

Several factors influence patient willingness to consider advance directives. Not everyone wishes to be involved in all choices.[21] Some elderly people appear to prefer surrogate decision making. Cultural perspectives regarding the importance of autonomy differ. Disenfranchised persons may fear inadequate treatment if an advance directive is present. Advance directives may also lack the requisite specificity to provide guidance to health care providers. Lawyers may advise clients of the advisability of advance directives during estate planning but have little expertise in describing or understanding medical conditions and technology. Hospital admissions, already stressful, involve multiple consent forms; advance directives information may be misplaced or not fully understood. (It has been suggested that advance directives materials be mailed to patients 1 week before anticipated admission to obtain a greater response rate.[22]) In addition, many physicians are unwilling to broach the subject of advance directives, perhaps fearing diminished authority or undermining of the physician-patient relationship.

Societally, there is a lack of consensus regarding many important questions about end-of-life decision making. What factors justify overriding an advance directive?[23] What weight should be given to the interests of others, such as family members, caretakers, and society in general? What safeguards should be put in place to ensure that patients are not coerced into signing advance directives?

Do-Not-Resuscitate Orders

Refusal to follow a DNR order or placing an individual on life support systems against his or her express wishes may constitute a battery.[24] This is a legal term for nonconsensual touching and has been used in cases alleging lack of informed consent. Plaintiffs have also been successful bringing such suits on a negligence theory. However, courts have generally declined to recognize a cause of action for "wrongful living."[25]

Hospitals may be asked to pay for care provided after a patient or family has requested removal of treatment. In a New York case, a court determined that the family remained liable for medical bills as the patient's wishes and New York law were too obscure at the time to permit removal of life support.[26] In general, life supports may be withdrawn without judicial procedure, considering family wishes to be conclusive, but if the institution is uncertain or if family members disagree, an institution is within its rights to refuse to withdraw until it seeks judicial resolution.[27] Note, however, that families have sought to recover money damages when a patient is placed on life support in spite of a DNR order.

In general, criminal penalties have not been imposed for failure to follow a DNR order, although several cases have been brought. In a 1983 California case, two physicians were prosecuted for murder for withdrawal of nutrition and hydration from a comatose patient, despite the consent of the patient's wife and children.[28] The court dismissed the case against the physicians.

According to one legal commentator, the legal risk for forcing an individual to receive medical intervention against his or her express wishes is greater than for withdrawing unwanted treatment (as expressed by a competent patient or through advanced directives).[29]

Another attorney wrote, "Because they fear liability, physicians and hospitals have sometimes been reluctant to follow the directives of patients and their families. While liability is theoretically possible, it is no more likely that physicians and other health care providers will be held liable for following treatment refusals than for their many other decisions and actions.... Exposure to civil liability is probably greater from refusing to honor the directives of the patient and the family."[30]

Health care providers should watch for legal warning signs—vacillation (by patients or family members regarding their wishes), dispute among family members, or uncertainty among medical staff—and may then wish to seek judicial intervention. Facilities must keep the interests of the patient primary.

Although right-to-die cases are typically the focus of discussion, reverse situations are beginning to appear. Hilda Wanglie was an 87-year-old woman who had a sudden onset cardiac arrest in 1991.[31, 32] She was in a persistent vegetative state, dependent on a ventilator and feeding tube. Eight months later, physicians declared her case to be futile and asked the court to permit respirator removal despite the family's objections. The court denied the request, affirming the right of family members to decide not to remove the ventilator.

There is no definitive legal precedent in the area of medical futility.[29] Cases are few; many hospital legal counsels continue to advise providing requested treatment, even if physicians consider doing so to be futile. However, a rising number of such cases can be anticipated given the shift in reimbursement incentives; although facilities were previously reimbursed for treatment, many health care plans' and diagnosis-related groups' approaches provide an incentive not to treat.

The notion of medical futility raises significant ethical and legal questions.[16] Who should decide that the situation is futile? What criteria should be used, and how should futility be defined? The picture is complicated by medical uncertainty and the conscious and subconscious value judgments health professionals and others may make, especially regarding the aged population. In reality, most physicians provide family or patient requested care due to fear of liability.

Physician-Assisted Suicide

On April 30, 1997, President Bill Clinton signed the Federal Assisted Suicide Funding Restriction Act of 1997 prohibiting the use of federal funds for physician-assisted suicide.[33] Prohibited by statute in most states,* physician-assisted suicide has become the subject of national debate. Michigan's Dr. Kevorkian has served jail time for assisting patient deaths.[34, 35] The Michigan court distinguishes between assisted suicide and withdrawal of life support—merely letting nature run its course.

In 1997, the U.S. Supreme Court upheld Washington and New York state bans on physician-assisted suicide.[36, 37] The Court looked to the United States' historical opposition to suicide in determining that plaintiffs did not have a constitutional liberty interest in an assisted suicide. Furthermore, the Court considered the states' interest in protecting vulnerable groups, such as the disabled, "from abuse, neglect and mistakes."[36] Finally, the Court noted the need to preserve the physician's traditional role as healer. The Court concluded that permitting removal of artificial life supports while banning physician-assisted suicide did not violate the equal protection clause or the due process clause of the U.S. Constitution.

Application to Case 5.2

Practically speaking, most patients and families do not litigate regarding provision of unconsented-to care. However, unconsented-to touching, including medical treatment, constitutes battery under the common law. Lillian and the facility may be liable for battery for providing unconsented-to treatment and perhaps for negligence. In addition, should Mrs. Poole die, her family may not pay for care provided after the resuscitation effort. Lillian might be subject to disciplinary action by the facility for failure to follow a written directive. It is possible that a state licensure board may consider her actions to be unprofessional conduct and thus grounds for discipline under the practice act.

ETHICAL ANALYSIS

From the ethical standpoint, Case 5.2 raises the question of when it is permissible to violate a patient's autonomy due to one's personal convictions. Implicitly, it raises the issue of how competing values should be arbitrated in a pluralistic society.

---

*For example, in Tennessee, assisted suicide is a Class D felony, carrying a penalty of 2–12 years' imprisonment and a $5,000 fine (Tennessee Code Annotated 39-13-216). Assisted suicide includes providing the means or intentionally participating in a physical act that directly and intentionally brings about another person's death.

The *Guide for Professional Conduct* [7] states that "PTs shall recognize that each individual is different from all other individuals and shall respect and be responsive to those differences" (1.1A) and that "PTs are to be guided at all times by concern for the physical, psychological, and socioeconomic welfare of those individuals entrusted to their care" (1.1B). This suggests that Lillian should have placed her patient's autonomy ahead of her own religious convictions. If Lillian felt strongly that she could not participate in Mrs. Poole's expressed decision, one of her options was to have someone else provide physical therapy for Mrs. Poole. However, these kinds of solutions are not always practical.

Other methods of dealing with conflicts of values are the use of an institutional ethics committee (IEC) or ethics consultation. More than 60% of hospitals with more than 200 beds have had IECs since 1986.[38, 39] IECs have been endorsed by the American Medical Association, the U.S. Department of Health and Human Services, and the President's Commission for the Study of Ethical Problems in Medicine and Biomedical and Behavioral Research. The JCAHO requires some method for dealing with ethical issues that arise in patient care.[39] IECs represent one method to meet this requirement. Some states, such as Maryland, have mandated hospitals to have IECs.[40] Ross and colleagues[41] pointed out that "ethics committees are popular in concept and controversial in practice. An understanding of the history, and particularly the origins, of the ethics committee movement might help committee members appreciate this paradox." The precursors of current IECs were

1. Committees that selected dialysis patients in the 1960s.
2. Prognosis committees, which developed in response to the Quinlan case. (The judge ordered that a committee convene to verify the prognosis given.)
3. Abortion selection committees before the 1973 legalization of abortion.
4. Medical-moral committees charged with assessing the compatibility of treatment with Catholic teachings in Catholic hospitals.
5. Institutional review boards formed in the 1970s to review all federally funded research (see Chapter 6).[41]

These committees had vastly different compositions, roles, and authority. In spite of the growing popularity and proliferation of IECs, they continue to assume diverse forms and models. An IEC is typically a multidisciplinary committee that performs the following three functions[41]:

1. Education of the members of the organization in ethical matters
2. Recommendation of policies and guidelines (historically they have focused on DNR policies)
3. Case review and consultation (the IEC may itself serve as a consultation team or may train other teams or individuals)

Beyond these basic functions, individual committees emphasize different portions of their responsibilities.

There are many unresolved questions regarding the role, authority, liability, and mechanisms of accountability of IECs. Are the decisions of the IEC binding? Are committee members legally liable for its decisions, or do committee members have immunity (a question that varies according to state law)?[39] Although some proponents argue for using IECs as an alternative to the courts, Fleetwood and Unger[39] noted that the following questions need to be addressed: "Several questions require close scrutiny in assessing whether ethics committees offer a reasonable alternative to the accepted option of judicial intervention. First, do committees follow a rigorous process? Second, are committee recommendations sound? Third, would immunity conferral serve patients' interests? Fourth, do committee consultations warrant the same legal authority as clinical consultations?" Given the diversity in existing IECs and the little that is known about them, it is not surprising to learn that Fleetwood and Unger thought that the answer to all of these questions is no. Three major problems are the inexperience of committee members (who are usually hospital employees), the lack of due process for patients, and the potential for conflict of interest for committee members.[39] Although Fleetwood and Unger's suggested qualifications would be good for all IECs, one wonders whether even judicial review would pass muster according to these criteria.

Although some IECs serve as ethics consultants within their institutions, many hospitals hire professionals trained in ethics to provide ethics consultation. Some consultants are trained in philosophy; others are health care professionals who have received further training in bioethics or medical ethics. Walker[42] noted that the discussion in ethics consultation has shifted from content issues and toward process issues:

> Literature of the last fifteen years [since the mid-1970s to mid-1980s] on moral expertise and ethics consulting shows a shift in emphasis from issues of content to those of process—from what the ethicist knows, to what the ethicist does or enables.

At the same time, the concept of the consultant's role has evolved from an engineer who analyzes ethical thought to a facilitator within an institutional context. The focus of discussion has shifted from thoughts and principles to matters of institutional context, accountability, and the relationship of moral deliberation within hospitals to society at large.[42]

A study at one institution demonstrated that, overall, physicians and nurses were more satisfied with clinical ethics consultation than were patients and family members.[43] Although 96% of the physicians and 95% of nurses thought that the consultation was helpful, only 65% of families found it helpful. Families who did not find the consultation helpful cited lack of communication between staff as a problem. This may support Walker's suggestion that the dual purpose of an ethics consultant is illustrated by the analogies of architect and mediator, whose role is to keep moral space open: "The ethicist's special responsibility is to keep open, accessible, and active (and, if necessary to create and design with others) those moral-reflective spaces in institutional life where a sound and shared process of deliberation and negotiation can go on."[42]

Case 5.3 is based on the real case of Don Cowart.[44] Don was severely burned when his truck's carburetor ignited propane gas from a gas leak. His father was killed in the blast. Don sustained numerous injuries including extensive burns, loss of vision, and injuries to his arms and legs. He was hospitalized for 14 months. Throughout this period, he requested permission to end treatment and to die. Later, he changed his name to Dax, completed law school, and began advocating for patient's rights.

CASE 5.3

Robert Hoadie is a 30-year-old man who sustained severe deep thickness burns over 98% of his body. He was working on his truck when the gas tank ignited and blew up. Before the accident, Robert was an avid hiker and outdoorsman. His vocation is the ministry; he serves a small rural Methodist church. He is single and has no significant other in his life. Since the accident, Robert has consistently requested that his doctor permit him to die. He states that God would not want him to have to live like this and he is prepared to "go to God." He believes that the hospital is artificially prolonging his life. You are working in the burn unit and your job is to provide hydrotherapy, debridement, and exercise to prevent contractures. Robert daily pleads with you to stop treatment, stating that you are violating his rights by taking him to the tub room.

QUESTIONS AND NOTES FOR FURTHER REFLECTION

1. Use the four principles and the APTA guides to analyze Case 5.3.

2. You are an ethics consultant or part of an IEC that has been called to consult. How will you function? Remember the dis-

tinction between content and process. What will you do to facilitate "keeping moral space open." With whom will you talk?

3. Does this case meet Miller's four senses of autonomy (see Chapter 2)?

4. What are the appropriate role and authority of IECs? What are the appropriate limitations on their authority?

5. Consider the application of the legal principles of battery (unconsented-to touching) to Case 5.3. Recall also that the Supreme Court in the Cruzan case stated that "a competent person has a constitutionally protected liberty interest in refusing unwanted medical treatment."[12]

CASE 5.4

Ryan Caldwell is a PT for ABC Rehabilitation Company. He has been sent to evaluate several newly admitted patients at an extended care facility with which his company has a contract. Mr. Blevins is a 75-year-old man with Parkinson's disease and schizophrenia. He had been living with his daughter until 2 weeks ago, when he fell at home. Ryan has been asked to assess Mr. Blevins' overall mobility and to make recommendations regarding assistive device versus wheelchair use. Following his assessment, Ryan finds that Mr. Blevins is unsafe to ambulate independently but that he is able to walk with a rolling walker with minimum-to-moderate assistance for approximately 50 feet. He recommends that the nursing staff walk Mr. Blevins to the bathroom (rather than providing a urinal) and that Mr. Blevins be walked to the community dining hall instead of eating meals in his room. The nursing supervisor tells Ryan that she does not have the staff to sustain this level of activity with Mr. Blevins; she asserts that he is very confused and his physical abilities decline when he refuses his medication. She believes that he is at risk for falls and should be kept in a Posey restraint in the chair at all times.

LEGAL ANALYSIS: USE OF RESTRAINTS

Recognizing the detrimental physical, cognitive, and social effects of restraint use,* Congress enacted legislation within the Omnibus Bud-

---

*Detrimental effects include decreased mobility, leading to further balance, strength, and range of motion deficits; general deconditioning; skin problems; incontinence; decreased appetite and possible dehydration; increased cardiac and respiratory problems; depression; increased agitation; humiliation; fear; cognitive decline; and the risk of strangulation by improper restraint application.[45–48]

get Reconciliation Act (OBRA) to limit inappropriate use of restraining devices.[49]

Under OBRA, a nursing facility must protect and promote the rights of each resident, including

> (ii) The right to be free from physical or mental abuse, corporal punishment, involuntary seclusion, and any physical or chemical restraints imposed for the purposes of discipline or convenience and not required to treat the resident's medical symptoms. Restraints may only be imposed
>
> (I) to ensure the physical safety of the resident or other residents, and only on the written order of a physician that specifies the duration and circumstances under which the restraints are to be used (except in emergency circumstances ... until such an order could reasonably be obtained).
>
> [Physical restraints include] [a]ny manual method of physical or mechanical device, material, or equipment attached or adjacent to the resident's body that the individual cannot move easily which restricts free movement or normal access to one's body. Leg restraints, arm restraints, hand mitts, soft ties or vests, wheelchair safety bars, and Geri-chairs *are* physical restraints.[50]

Some states have further statutory protections for extended care facility residents. Tennessee law requires that a patient under restraint be checked every 30 minutes; every 2 hours the restraints should be released, the patient's position changed, and the patient should be exercised.[51] In some states, inappropriate use of restraints is classified as a form of criminal elder abuse, with substantial penalties for perpetrators.

Penalties for failure to comply with federal law, as enforced through state-conducted facility surveys, include decertification from participation in Medicare and Medicaid and restrictions on Medicare admissions and fines. Under OBRA, the facility is responsible for medical care decisions. The presence of a physician's order may not excuse a facility for improper restraint usage.

Restraints are often used by providers who fear liability associated with falls and believe restraint reduction will increase staffing costs. This appears to be unfounded, as shown in both the medical literature and case law. Studies have shown that no increase in nursing care is required when a restraint reduction program is instituted.[48]

Some studies suggest that restraint usage has diminished significantly since OBRA was enacted: One shows a decrease in the percentage of patients restrained from 41% in 1988 to 22% in 1992[47]; another study suggests that from 1989 to 1991, usage dropped by 47%.[52] Studies differ, however, in their definitions of restraint (e.g., whether such items as side rails and lap trays are considered restraints).

Legal Intervention

There have been no reported cases as of this writing at the federal appellate level regarding enforcement of the OBRA restraint provisions.

The general legal principle is to look to the industry standard in determining whether an individual or a facility has been negligent—that is, did this person act in a manner consistent with the actions of a reasonably prudent PT in a similar situation? To the extent that the restraint guidelines have reduced use of restraints (or at least have increased consideration and monitoring of restraint usage), it may be increasingly difficult for facilities to show that they were following industry standards in restraining a particular patient.

The restraint use standard for extended care facilities is distinguishable from that for an acute care facility; there are no federal guidelines for acute care. The usual presumption in the hospital environment is that agents of the hospital can use restraints as needed due to the severity of the acute illness and the unfamiliar and temporary surroundings. Courts look to the foreseeability of the injury (e.g., medications administered, history of prior falls, general physical and cognitive functioning, age, and physical environment) in determining whether the facility acted reasonably.

In a 1948 case, a 26-year-old man was admitted with pneumonia, a spiking fever, and delirium to an acute care facility.[53] The family had asked to remain with the patient or to have a private nurse in the room with the patient. The patient was restrained in bed with leather wrist and leg restraints; he unfastened these and jumped out of the third floor window, dying from cerebral hemorrhage several hours later. Liability was imposed on the hospital as the fall was considered reasonably foreseeable. *Wooten v. United States* involved an 83-year-old man admitted to a hospital with an acute myocardial infarction.[54] His wife had asked to stay in the room with him. The patient fell, sustaining a severe head injury. The court found the hospital liable, as the patient's age, medication, and general condition permitted facility staff to foresee the situation. Compare this case with *White v. Baptist Memorial Hospital,*[55] in which no recovery was awarded with an unforeseeable fall.

Although it remains somewhat unclear in the literature whether an increase in falls is a predictable effect of restraint reduction programs, some evidence suggests that restraints do not increase serious fall-related injuries.[56] Regarding falls and potential falls, courts look to the foreseeability of the fall in judging the appropriateness of the facility's actions, again in accordance with the prevailing standard. In general, extended care facilities are much less likely to be sued than acute care facilities. One study showed that one-fourth of extended care facility lawsuits involved falls. Of these, 25% alleged negligent supervision, 10% cited failure to restrain, and 5% cited failure to use bed rails.[48]

As one legal analyst who focuses on this area stated, adverse suits are successful only when it can be shown that there is a failure to provide for a resident's safety, as evidenced through a pattern of improperly assessing a resident's needs, failure to properly monitor or supervise a resident, failure to respond to a fall or to wandering in a timely and professionally acceptable manner, or staff conduct endangering a resident. "Any legal exposure associated with failure to restrain residents is outweighed by the legal risks attached to the improper application of physical restraints.... [M]ounting data show that physical restraints used in the name of defensive medicine may not only fail to be defensive, but may actually be counterproductive."[56]

The following are some suggestions for a facility to manage risks associated with restraint use.

1.   Obtain consent from the patient or surrogate for the use of restraints (or non-use if facility recommends them). The patient must be informed of the symptoms necessitating use of restraints, of how restraints will optimize physical and psychosocial well-being, and of the adverse effects of restraints. This process shifts risk to patient or family member. Note, however, that a resident's consent to the use of a restraint does not relieve a facility from liability if the restraint is improperly applied.*

2.   Develop a process for resolving disputes between the facility and resident or surrogate or among staff and family members.

3.   Institute policies evincing a preference for the least restrictive restraint alternative; make current and prospective patients and families aware of the policies.

4.   Educate staff regarding the policies and safe restraint usage. There must be facility involvement and support at all levels, including the governing body and physicians.

5.   Enforce the policies (including imposing disciplinary action against individuals in violation).

6.   Establish a restraint monitoring schedule and documentation (e.g., cushion color changes to indicate that a resident has been repositioned, a schedule for taking the patient to the toilet).

7.   Institute procedures to obtain physician's written orders as soon as possible after emergency application of restraints.

8.   Monitor all restraints routinely. Include documentation of side effects, assessment of ongoing need, and full reassessment with any signs of deterioration.

---

*See *Bauman v. Seven Acres Jewish Geriatric Center*, no. 86-44019 (234th Dist. Ct. Tex. 1990) and *Davis v. Montrose Bay Care Center* (June 19, 1989), cases involving strangulation by restraining vests. In the Bauman case, the jury awarded $4.4 million in compensatory damages and $35 million in punitive damages. These amounts were later set aside due to misconduct by the plaintiff's attorneys and settled under undisclosed terms.

9. Create an interdisciplinary restraint committee to review restraint needs; committee members should become familiar with fall reduction literature.

10. Create an individualized restraint plan for each resident, documenting thoroughly specific reasons for their use.

The following are some suggestions for a practicing PT to promote restraint reduction:

1. Advocate for additional services as warranted to reduce risk of falls: day program activities, PT or occupational therapist services, exercise classes, behavior modification activities, rocking chairs, soothing music, recliners for agitated residents, or naps to prevent overfatigue.
2. Educate management about commercially available or easily fabricated restraint alternatives.
3. Participate in development of restraint alternatives and offer to serve on the restraint committee.

PTs may be in a unique role to make recommendations regarding the physical environment of patients to optimize safe mobility and limit fall risk. Options include placing a resident's mattress on the floor, using campus security systems, recommending appropriate lighting and floor surfaces, providing a safe area for wanderers, and conducting thorough seating assessments.

Application to Case 5.4

The case of Mr. Blevins is the type of situation that the OBRA requirements were designed to combat—that is, physical restraints imposed for the purposes of discipline or convenience and not required to treat the resident's medical symptoms. Numerous other initiatives should be explored to ensure Mr. Blevins' safety while permitting movement. In the event that the facility follows the nursing supervisor's recommendations, it must be able to show that it acted to ensure Mr. Blevins' physical safety, and the restraint must be ordered and the orders regularly updated by a physician. Failure to follow these requirements may result in decertification, restrictions on Medicare admissions, and fines.

Additionally, the facility may be liable under state statutes governing nursing home restraint usage. If the restraint is applied improperly and injury to Mr. Blevins occurs, the facility could be liable for failure to adequately train staff and for negligence. Furthermore, in some states, inappropriate restraint usage is classified as a form of criminal elder abuse, subjecting staff to criminal penalties.[57, 58] (See Greenberg[59] for additional resources.)

NOTES AND QUESTIONS FOR FURTHER REFLECTION

1. Use the four principles (autonomy, beneficence, nonmalefi-cence, and justice) to analyze Case 5.4.

2. Use a virtue-based approach to ethical analysis of Case 5.4.

REFERENCES

1. S.1360.
2. Smith Hurd Annot. 410 ILCS 305/1 et seq.
3. *Tarrant County Hospital District v. Hughes*, 734 S.W.2d 675 (Tex. Ct. App. 1987).
4. D.C. Code §2-3305.14 (a)(16).
5. Hawaii Statutes Annotated 461J-12(a)(2).
6. *Rost v. State Bd of Psychology*, 659 A.2d 626 (Pa. Comwlth. 1995).
7. American Physical Therapy Association. Guide for Professional Conduct. Alexandria, VA: American Physical Therapy Association, 1997.
8. Joint Commission on Accreditation of Healthcare Organizations. Comprehensive Accreditation Manual for Hospitals. Oak Brook Terrace, IL: Joint Commission on Accreditation of Healthcare Organizations, 1994.
9. Ubel PA, Zell MM, Miller DJ, et al. Elevator talk: observational study of inappropriate comments in a public space. Am J Med 1995;99:190.
10. Woodward B. The computerized-based patient record and confidentiality. N Engl J Med 1995;333:1419.
11. *In re Quinlan*, 70 N.J. 10, 355 A.2d 647, *cert denied*, 429 U.S. 922 (1976).
12. *Cruzan v. Director, Missouri Department of Health*, 110 S.Ct. 2841, 497 U.S. 261 (1990).
13. *Cruzan v. Harman*, 760 S.W.2d 408 (Mo. 1988).
14. 42 U.S.C.S. 1395 cc(f) (1992).
15. Teno J, Lindemann Nelson H, Lynn J. Advance care planning: priorities for ethical and empirical research. Hastings Center Report 1994;24:S32.
16. Danis M. Following advance directives. Hastings Center Report 1994;24:S21.
17. Danis M, Southerland L, Garrett J. A prospective study of advance directives for life-sustaining care. N Engl J Med 1991;324:882.
18. Sugarman J. Recognizing good decision making for incapacitated patients. Hastings Center Report 1994;24:S11.
19. Cohen-Mansfield J, Rabinovich B, Lipson S, et al. The decision to execute a durable power of attorney for health care and preferences regarding the utilization of life-sustaining treatments in nursing home residents. Arch Intern Med 1991;151:289.
20. Emanuel L, Barry M, Stoeckle J. Advance directives for medical care—a case for greater use. N Engl J Med 1991;324:889.
21. Wetle T. Individual preferences and advance directives. Hastings Center Report 1994;24:S5.

22. Silverman H, Fry S, Armistead N. Nurses' perspectives on implementation of the patient self-determination act. J Clin Ethics 1994;5:30.

23. Brock D. Good decisionmaking for incompetent patients. Hastings Center Report 1994;24:S8.

24. *Anderson v. St. Francis-St. George Hosp.*, 83 Ohio App.3d 221, 614 N.E.2d 841 (1992); *rev. denied*, 66 Ohio St.3d 1459, 610 N.E.2d 423; *appeal after remand*, 671 N.E.2d 225 (1995); *Estate of Leach v. Shapiro*, 13 Ohio App.3d 393, 469 N.E.2d 1047 (1984).

25. *Benoy v. Simons*, 66 Wash. App. 56, 831 P.2d 167; *rev. denied*, 120 Wash. 2d 1014, 844 P.2d 435 (1992).

26. *Grace Plaza v. Elbaum*, 82 N.Y.2d 10, 603 N.Y.S.2d 386, 623 N.E.2d 513 (1993).

27. *Ross v. Hilltop Rehabilitation Hosp.*, 124 F.R.D. 660, 676 F. Suppl. 528 (1988).

28. *Barber v. Superior Court*, 147 Cal. App. 3d 1006, 195 Cal. Rptr. 484 (2d Dist. 1983).

29. Kapp M. Geriatrics and the Law. New York: Springer, 1992.

30. Miller R. Problems in Health Care Law. Gaithersburg, MD: Aspen, 1996.

31. Angell M. The case of Helga Wanglie: a new kind of "right to die" case. N Engl J Med 1991;325:511.

32. Miles SH. Informed demand for non-beneficial medical treatment. N Engl J Med 1991;325:512.

33. 42 U.S.C. §14401 et seq.

34. *Kevorkian v. Thompson*, 947 F. Suppl. 1152 (Ed. Mich. 1997).

35. *People v. Kevorkian*, 447 Mich. 436, 527 N.W.2d 714 (1994).

36. *Washington v. Glucksberg*, 65 U.S.L.W. 4669 (1997).

37. *Vacco v. Quill*, 65 U.S.L.W. 4695 (1997).

38. Gibson JM, Kushner TK. Will the "conscience of an institution" become society's servant? Hastings Center Report 1986;16:9.

39. Fleetwood J, Unger SS. Institutional ethics committees and the shield of immunity. Ann Intern Med 1994;120:320, 322.

40. Maryland Health-General Code Annotated §19-370-374.

41. Ross JW, Glaser JW, Rasiniski-Gregory D, et al. Health Care Ethics Committees: The Next Generation. Chicago: American Hospital Publishing, 1993.

42. Walker MU. Keeping moral space open: new images of ethics consulting. Hastings Center Report 1993;23:33, 37.

43. McClung JA, Kamer RS, DeLuca M, Barber HJ. Evaluation of a medical ethics consultation service: opinions of patients and health care providers. Am J Med 1996;100:456.

44. Arras JD, Steinbock B. Ethical Issues in Modern Medicine (4th ed). Mountain View, CA: Mayfield Publishing, 1995;195.

45. 42 U.S.C. §1396r(c)(1)(A)(ii).

46. Egbebike J. Complying with OBRA: Managing Restraint Reduction Programs in Nursing Homes and Healthcare Centers. Old Bridge, NJ: PTS Publishing, 1993.

47. Ejaz F, Folmar S, Kaufmann M. Restraint reduction: can it be achieved? Gerontologist 1994;34:694.

48. Evans L, Strumpf N. Tying down the elderly: a review of the literature on physical restraint J Am Geriatr Soc 1989;37:65.

49. Miles S, Meyers R. Untying the elderly: 1989 to 1993. Update. Clin Geriatr Med 1994;10:513.

50. Health Care Financing Administration. Medicaid State Operations Manual (Interpretive Guidelines for February 2, 1989; Transmittal 232, Sept. 1989); Washington, DC: U.S. Dept. of Health and Human Services.
51. Tennessee Code Annotated 68-11-803 (c)(3).
52. Mion LC, Mercurio AT. Methods to reduce restraints: process, outcomes, and future directions. J Gerontol Nurs 1992;18:5.
53. *Spivey v. St. Thomas Hospital*, 211 S.W.2d 450 (1947).
54. 574 F. Supp. 200 (1982), affirmed 722 F.2d 743 (1983).
55. 363 F.2d 37 (1966).
56. Kapp M. Nursing home restraints and legal liability. J Legal Med 1992;13:1.
57. Cal. Wel. and Inst. Code Ann. 15610(c)(6) & 15632 (West Supp. 1990).
58. 1990 R.I. Pub. Laws §23-17.8-1(e).
59. Greenberg R. OBRA's challenge to physical therapy: find alternatives to physical restraints. PT Bull 1996;11:11.

6

Research and Educational Issues

This chapter addresses legal and ethical issues encountered in the educational arena. Ethical and legal dimensions of the research process have become increasingly important, especially following discovery of unethical practices during the second World War. The result has been the gradual increase in standards for and public awareness of the protection of human subjects. One of the cases in this chapter addresses legal and ethical problems encountered in research. At the heart of legal and ethical aspects of research is the concept of informed consent. A basic definition is offered, the history of the concept is outlined, and emerging trends are discussed. Federal guidelines for research are also described. Some of the challenges caused by the introduction of business principles and management to health care were discussed in Chapter 3. A business environment adds even more complexity to the clinical education arena. Four of the cases in this chapter discuss legal and ethical issues in the area of clinical education.

CASE 6.1

Meyer Livingston is a physical therapist (PT) who has just started the Ph.D. program in biomechanics at a prominent university. Since graduating from PT school, Meyer has dreamed of completing a doctoral program and teaching physical therapy. As part of his stipend, Meyer has been assigned to assist Dr. Alfred Nickerson with research. Dr. Nickerson has been one of the most productive researchers on the faculty and has been awarded numerous grants.

Dr. Nickerson is currently pursuing a large private grant. At the first meeting to discuss Meyer's role in the research process, they discuss the details of the project. Dr. Nickerson gives Meyer a prospectus of the study, which will involve human subjects. The prospectus does not include the application for review by the institutional review board (IRB), so Meyer asks Dr. Nickerson if

IRB approval has already been obtained. Dr. Nickerson says, "You have a lot to learn about this process, Meyer. I used to try to jump through all those hoops, but the university was so slow to process my application that I'd never get any grant money if I waited for them. Besides, the proposal calls for obtaining informed consent from the participants. The secretary will take care of all of that."

Meyer is concerned by the conversation. University guidelines state that all research must be approved by the appropriate review committee. However, Dr. Nickerson is famous for carrying grudges. Meyer fears that speaking up about this issue might ruin his chances of ever receiving his Ph.D.

RESEARCH PROPOSAL REVIEW

Although Meyer is unsure about the ethical obligations involved in private research, he knows that all federal research proposals involving human subjects must be submitted to an IRB. This is necessary both ethically and legally. Federal law requires that research conducted with human subjects be approved by an IRB.[1] The IRB must review the research proposal and assess (among other things) risk to subjects as well as adequacy of informed consent. This legal requirement reflects the growing public consensus regarding the rights and protection of human subjects. Review boards were designed to guarantee these rights, which are captured by the concepts of informed consent and protection of human subjects. An understanding of the historical development of the concept of informed consent and protection of human subjects provides insight into the ethical dimensions of Meyer's dilemma.

INFORMED CONSENT IN THE RESEARCH SETTING

Historical Perspective

The notions of informed consent and protection of human subjects have been in evolution in American medicine and in society at large since 1957. Although it may seem that current standards for informed consent have always been a part of health care delivery, the fact is that accepted standards for informed consent are relatively new. In a now-classic 1978 article about informed consent in medical treatment, Jay Katz[2] noted that the notion of informed consent is more a legal than a medical concept. Indeed, Katz called informed consent a concept alien to medical practice. He drew two conclusions about the interplay between legal and ethical aspects of informed consent.

> Two significant conclusions can be drawn: (1) "informed consent" is a creature of law and not a medical prescription. A duty to inform patients has never been promulgated by the medical profession.... (2) When judges were confronted with claims of lack of informed consent, no medical precedent, no medical position papers, and no analytic medical thinking existed on this subject. Thus physicians were ill prepared to shape judges' notions on informed consent with thoughtful and systematic positions of their own.[2]

Beauchamp and Childress[3] noted that the term *informed consent* did not appear until 10 years after the Nuremberg Trials exposed medical experimental atrocities perpetrated on human subjects by the Nazis. Although informed consent serves the dual purposes of preventing harm (nonmaleficence) and preserving autonomy, there has been an increasing tendency in biomedical ethics to view informed consent primarily from the perspective of autonomy.[3] Some writers see this change as indicative of a shift in the perspective of biomedical ethics and society in general to be dominated by autonomy and individual rights.[3] Indeed, it has been suggested that the current period represents a time in which concern for autonomy is seriously out of balance with concerns for beneficence[4] (including beneficence directed toward societal goals).

This shift toward an autonomy-based understanding of informed consent is due in part to a number of highly publicized studies in which the rights of human subjects were clearly violated. Many of these resulted in the promulgation of a new code or standard.* Some examples of higher standards or laws for protecting subjects that resulted from improperly performed research are:

1.   The Nuremberg Code (1947): Revelations about World War II atrocities resulted in formulation of the Nuremberg Code, which outlined 10 principles to govern medical research. The Nuremberg Code contained the basic components of informed consent: (a) voluntary consent, (b) disclosure of risks, (c) avoiding pain and suffering, (d) right of the subject to terminate, (e) balancing of risks and benefits, and (f) the responsibility of the researcher. The importance of the Nurem-

---

*This history is detailed in the Report of the Advisory Committee on Human Radiation Experimentation (ACHRE). This account is based on the history contained in that report. All information was obtained from the ACHRE report obtained via the Internet through the U.S. Department of Energy at http://www.tis.eh.doe.gov/systems/hrad. This information is also available at http://www.seas.gwu.edu/nsarchive/radiation or through the U.S. Government Printing Office.

berg Code is highlighted by Annas and Grodin[5] who noted that "all contemporary debate on human experimentation is grounded in Nuremberg."

2.   Declaration of Helsinki: Adopted by the World Medical Association in 1964, the Declaration of Helsinki differentiated research within a therapeutic context from nontherapeutic research. (The declaration was revised in 1975, 1983, and 1989.)[6]

3.   The National Research Act of 1974: The National Research Act of 1974 established the National Commission for the Protection of Human Subjects of Biomedical and Behavioral Research and endorsed the regulations of the U.S. Department of Health, Education and Welfare (HEW) (now the U.S. Department of Health and Human Services [HHS]). These regulations require that institutions seeking HEW grants establish a committee (later, IRB) to review grant applications to HEW.[7] This legislation came about in part as a result of the 40-year (1932–1972) Tuskegee experiments, in which treatment was withheld from African-American men with syphilis so the disease could be studied.

4.   The Belmont Report (1979): The Belmont Report is the report of a national committee commissioned in the National Research Act of 1974. During its 4 years of deliberation, the commission studied the issues of informed consent, autonomy, and other topics related to ethical research. The principles underlying the Belmont Report became famous as described by the ACHRE: "In the course of its deliberations, the commission identified three general moral principles—respect for persons, beneficence, and justice—as the appropriate framework for guiding the ethics of research involving human subjects. These three are known as the *Belmont principles* because they appeared in the Belmont Report...."[7]

5.   1980–1983 President's Committee for the Study of Ethical Problems in Medicine and Biomedical and Behavioral Research[7]: This commission recommended that the regulations formulated for HEW (now HHS) be applied to all federally funded research.

6.   1991 Adoption of the Common Rule: The Common Rule laid out the rules that apply to all federally funded research. "The rule directs a research institution to assure the federal government that it will provide and enforce protections for human subjects of research conducted under its auspices. These institutional assurances constitute the basic framework within which federal protections are effected. Local research institutions remain largely responsible for carrying out the specific directives of the Common Rule."[7]

The ACHRE describes the elements of informed consent as stipulated in the Common Rule as follows:

1. A statement that the study involves research, an explanation of the purposes of the research, and a description of the procedures to be followed
2. A description of any reasonably foreseeable risks or discomforts to the subject
3. A description of any benefits to the subjects or to others that might reasonably be expected
4. A disclosure of alternative procedures or courses of treatment
5. A statement describing the extent to which confidentiality of records identifying the subject will be maintained
6. For research involving more than minimal risk, an explanation of the availability and nature of any compensation or medical treatment if injury occurs
7. Identification of whom to contact for further information about subjects' rights and whom to contact in the event of a research-related injury
8. A statement that participation is voluntary, that refusal to participate will involve no penalty or loss of benefits to which the subject is otherwise entitled, and that the subject may discontinue participation at any time[7]

Although the Common Rule provides excellent procedures to provide disclosure, the availability of good procedures does not necessarily meet the requirement for informed consent from an ethical standpoint. According to Beauchamp and Childress,[3] informed consent should contain the following elements.

Threshold elements (preconditions)
   1.   Competence (to understand and decide)
   2.   Voluntariness (in deciding)
Information elements
   1.   Disclosure (of material information)
   2.   Recommendation (of a plan)
   3.   Understanding (of disclosure and information)
Consent elements
   1.   Decision (in favor of a plan)
   2.   Authorization (of the chosen plan)

If Beauchamp and Childress' elements of informed consent are compared to the elements of the Common Rule, it is seen that the latter emphasizes disclosure of information.[3] While disclosure of information is a necessary part of the process of informed consent, fulfillment of the other portions of informed consent depends in part on the sincere efforts of the researcher. Disclosure is a necessary but not sufficient part of informed consent.

The limitations of procedures to guarantee disclosure of information are well illustrated by the radiation experiments performed on human subjects during the Cold War. These experiments were performed to further medical and scientific knowledge. Does scientific and medical progress present an incentive to the researcher to downplay the risks to the subject? In the 1970s, Jay Katz, a medical ethicist, served as a member of the advisory committee that investigated the Tuskegee experiments. Katz also served on the ACHRE during 1994.[8] The proceedings of this committee provide an excellent review of the conduct of experiments on human subjects. The committee concluded that, in spite of the fact that standards for obtaining informed consent were available, radiation experiments were performed on human subjects during the Cold War without informed consent.

The comments of Jay Katz are more critical of the informed consent process than those of the committee as a whole, understandable in light of his personal involvement in investigating breaches of ethics spanning several decades. In a statement to the committee, he presented the following conclusions:

(1) In the quest to advance medical science, too many citizen-patients continue to serve, as they did during the Cold War period, as means for the sake of others.

(2) The length to which physician-investigators must go to seek "informed consent" remains sufficiently ambiguous so that patient-subjects' understandings of the consequences of their participation in research is all too often compromised.

(3) The resolution of the tensions inherent in the conduct of research—i.e., respect for citizen-patients' rights to, and interest in, self-determination on the one hand and the imperative to advance medical science, on the other—confronts government officials with policy choices that they were unwilling to address in any depth during the Cold War or for that matter in today's world.

(4) Our Recommendations only touch on these problems and at times make too much of the safeguards that have been introduced since 1974. The present regulatory process is flawed. It invites in subtle, but real, ways repetitions of the dignitary insults which unconsenting citizen-patients suffered during the Cold War.[8]

The American Physical Therapy Association (APTA) has published *Guidelines for Integrity in Physical Therapy Research* BOD 03-92-21-67. This document contains many of the elements found in other research codes. The guidelines state that researchers should comply with laws and regulations relating to research. The IRB is to review the research proposal and assess (among other things) risk to subjects as well as adequacy of informed consent.

The IRB process represents a minimal fulfillment of the informed consent process, fulfilling only what Beauchamp and Childress described as *information elements.*[3] The review by an objective board helps researchers to ensure that their personal investment in the research process does not prevent obtaining informed consent and disclosing both the risks and benefits of the experiment.

Application to Case 6.1

Meyer is in a difficult situation. To participate in the study may be illegal and unethical. Yet Meyer thinks that his future and his own self-interest may conflict with his legal and ethical obligations. How should he resolve the situation?

QUESTIONS AND NOTES FOR FURTHER REFLECTION

1. What are the barriers to obtaining informed consent in the research context?

2. What minimal conditions must be met to have obtained informed consent?

3. What should members of an IRB look for to determine that subjects do not feel pressured by medical providers to participate in research?

4. What process should private institutions that do not receive federal funds use in evaluating research proposals?

5. What are the ramifications of Dr. Nickerson's plan to have the secretary obtain informed consent? Which of Beauchamp and Childress' seven elements of informed consent are fulfilled by this process?

INFORMED CONSENT IN THE CLINICAL EDUCATION SETTING

Although it might seem logical that there should be very little difference between informed consent in experimental research and in treatment, there are important differences in the way that informed consent is viewed in the two arenas. One important difference is the relationship between patient and therapist in these settings.

The cases in this section deal with students who encounter ethical situations or dilemmas in the clinical education setting. The clinical education setting presents challenges for legal and ethical analysis in that the student is still training to assume a professional role. In addition to this status, students are subject to the power that the clinical instructor, the school, and the facility may wield over them. Specifically, students could be described as not being fully autonomous in clinical and ethical matters. They are particularly vulnerable to being in a situation that Purtilo[9] described as *ethical distress*. That is, they know the right thing to do but they are not empowered to do it.

Definition

Informed consent has been defined as an exchange of information between a therapist and a patient that enables a patient to make an informed choice about treatment options. The basis of informed consent is the patient's right of self-determination—that is, the right to make decisions about what happens to one's body. Informed consent should not be viewed by the therapist merely as a form to be completed, but rather as a substantive, ongoing dialogue with the patient that reflects changes in the therapeutic regimen and anticipated outcomes.

Liability

A few words about liability issues in the context of clinical education are in order before proceeding to the cases. Recall that a health care professional's actions are based on the prevailing standard of care. There is no special standard of care governing student conduct.

Clinical affiliation agreements may assign liability between the site and the school. However, in certain situations, liability may attach regardless of the specifics of the agreement. For example, a school can be found liable if it assigns a student to a clinical facility knowing that the student is not prepared to handle the patient load and patient injury results.[10] If a clinical instructor is uncertain of a student's ability to perform a particular procedure, he or she should assess the student's competency before assigning the task.

When a supervisor cosigns the note of a student, he or she becomes liable for the assessment and care provided to the patient.[11] Negligent supervision may in itself be actionable and may under some circumstances constitute aiding the unlicensed practice of physical therapy, a practice act violation in many states. If an instructor gives a student inappropriate instructions, the instructor may be held liable for student actions.[10]

Students must be clearly identified as such to enable patients to give true, adequate informed consent. Furthermore, failure to inform the patient that a student is involved in treatment can give rise to claims of fraud, deceit, misrepresentation, invasion of privacy, and breach of confidentiality.[10] Students can be held liable for intentional conduct such as battery, defamation, invasion of privacy, or sexual harassment.[10]

CASE 6.2

Tom Feingold is a student PT in a busy outpatient surgery clinic. During his affiliation with the clinic, Tom was assigned to perform evaluation and treatment of Bob Burkhardt. Bob had sustained a partial tear of his rotator cuff while playing tennis. Bob's orthopedic surgeon performed arthroscopic surgery. The operative notes state that the rotator cuff was badly frayed. The surgeon debrided the cuff and referred him for physical therapy. Tom treated Bob with the standard rotator cuff exercises. Three weeks following surgery, Bob experienced a pop while performing resistive exercise with an elastic band. He sued for professional negligence and asserted that he was never informed of the potential for reinjury. Tom's documentation contains no mention of his discussion with the patient of the risks of treatment. What legal and ethical issues are raised in this case?

LEGAL ANALYSIS

Legal Intervention

Informed consent is required by law under some state statutes, such as malpractice statutes.* In other states, informed consent has been developed through case law. In addition, informed consent is mandated by the Joint Commission on Accreditation of Healthcare Organizations (JCAHO) and by the APTA, through the *Standards of Practice for Physical Therapy and the Accompanying Criteria*,[12] the *Guide for Professional Conduct*,[13] and the House of Delegates policies (see *Ethical Analysis* later in this chapter).

What should be included in informed consent? Before treatment, a patient must be advised of the type of treatment recommended, any material decisional risks involved, the expected benefits or goals of treatment, and available alternatives, if any. The information must be conveyed in language the patient can understand. Informed consent

---

*See, for example, Tennessee Code Annotated, 29-26-118.

should be obtained by the therapist rather than a surrogate to provide an opportunity for the patient to ask questions.

Two different standards exist regarding the information to be provided to patients in obtaining informed consent. The first is the professional standard—that is, sharing that information that other professionals would consider necessary to share. The second standard is called the lay standard and requires the therapist to consider the information that the patient would consider necessary to make an informed decision. The standard varies by state law, defined either through statute or case law. In general, the greater the severity of potential injury, the higher the likelihood that a court would require disclosure, even if the incidence of the risk is low.

A seminal case in this area is *Canterbury v. Spence*.[14] The case involved a 19-year-old postlaminectomy patient who fell getting out of bed and subsequently experienced a partial paralysis. It was unclear whether the fall caused the paralysis, but the court ruled that the physician had not adequately informed the patient of the 1% risk of partial paralysis inherent in the surgical procedure.

Exceptions

There are exceptions to the requirement of informed consent. The first involves an emergency situation; in such cases, it is important to document thoroughly the rationale for any treatment procedures selected. A second exception is called therapeutic privilege, a situation in which a health care provider (usually a physician) believes it to be in the patient's best interest not to be fully advised of adverse risks to prevent further health problems. A third exception to the requirement of informed consent is treatment of minors or incompetents, in which case informed consent must be obtained from a surrogate.

Documentation

How should informed consent be documented? Although many health care providers rely on the generic hospital consent form, these typically do not address specific procedures. A hospital consent form may provide warning of certain risks, such as falling or overexertion. A written entry may be made in the medical record. A consent checklist may also be developed, delineating the most common therapeutic interventions and associated risks and benefits.[15] An alternative is a procedures manual that describes the routine consent information provided; therapists can then document "informed consent obtained" in the medical record.

Any form of informed consent must be updated as treatment changes over the course of therapy. Treatment refusals must be carefully documented, especially repeated refusals or refusals of recommended equipment or follow-up care. The risks of treatment that were communicated to the patient must also be clearly documented. If consent to treatment is not obtained at all, proceeding with treatment constitutes a battery or nonconsensual touching.

The purposes of medical records include communicating with other health care professionals, monitoring quality of care, serving as a research and educational resource, and serving as a business or legal document. Some states have requirements about the contents of medical records, either by statute or regulation. In addition, private regulatory agencies, such as the JCAHO, may specify the contents of adequate documentation.

Incident reports alert management to potential safety problems, record important facts, and create a legal record. Incident reports are generally kept separate from the rest of the medical record. Courts are split as to the discoverability of incident reports—that is, whether a plaintiff may obtain them in the course of litigation. Some legal counsel advise that such reports be identified as quality assurance documents or state that they were prepared at the facility attorney's direction for litigation. In jurisdictions in which reports are discoverable, such a disclaimer may be insufficient, as incident reports are generally prepared well in advance of the filing of a lawsuit.

Many facilities are adopting a system of documentation by exception, in which a care pathway is established and only variances from the pathway are charted. This practice is legally recognized in businesses that always follow a particular practice and document only variations. Questions sometimes arise as to foreseeability and completeness when an individual is offered choices only from a predetermined list of variances that do not describe the situation. Any inconsistencies between the variance selected and written documentation is subject to question.

Common problems in documentation include failure to date or sign notes or to identify the patient. Vague terms, such as "tolerated treatment well," are often used. Many notes do not refer to functionally based goals; they may contain large amounts of clinical data, such as range of motion, edema, and strength, but fail to link data to functional impairments, an increasing focal point for insurers. Subjective, imprecise goals, such as "increase strength," "improve posture," or "decrease pain," are also problematic.[16] Errors in the medical record should not be erased or covered with correction fluid. Rather, draw a single line through the mistaken entry, write the word *error*, and initial and date it. Illegible notation provides little defense in the event of a lawsuit and creates an impression of a sloppy provider. The same is true of improper spelling, grammar, and abbreviations.

Sufficiency of documentation is critical; failure to document adequately can subject a therapist to a variety of sanctions. An Ohio therapist's license was suspended for 30 days for violating the state practice act after the therapist failed to maintain adequate patient records, including failing to identify and document each patient's precautions, special problems, contraindications, goals, anticipated progress, and plan for reevaluation.[17] In another case, a physician was removed from participation in the Medicaid program for 5 years for failure to maintain records sufficient to justify tests ordered or medications prescribed.[18]

Who owns medical records, the patient, the provider, or the facility? Who has access to such records? While state laws differ, most state laws provide that ownership of the medical record rests with the facility treating the patient. Patients and their authorized representatives generally have the right to receive a copy of their medical records on request.

How long should medical records be kept? Many states have statutes that specify the required retention period for medical records. In the absence of such a law, therapists should keep medical records for *at least* the period of the statute of limitations on personal injury cases (usually 1–5 years). Note that the statute of limitations for minors usually begins when they reach the age of majority. Therefore, pediatric records should be kept for 18 years plus the applicable statute of limitations period.

Application to Case 6.2

Case 6.2 points to the absolute need for adequate and clear documentation to support a therapist's position in defending a lawsuit. The medical record serves to jog the therapist's memory regarding information conveyed to a patient, as a case likely will not proceed to trial until several years after treatment. The record also verifies for the judge and jury that the therapist did what he or she says was done in conveying risks, benefits, and alternatives to a patient. In the case as presented, the jury must weigh the evidence as a whole and the credibility of witness testimony to determine whether adequate informed consent was obtained. Liability would also likely extend to the supervisor, who presumably cosigned the note and supervised the student's clinical performance.

ETHICAL ANALYSIS

There is an intrinsic difference in the relationship between the therapist as clinician and the therapist as researcher. In the therapeutic relationship, the goal is the health of the patient. On the other hand, the goal in research is the betterment of society as a whole through increasing knowledge.[19] Both goals to some degree come under the rubric of beneficence, but the goals imply a very different relationship with the patient.

The *Code of Ethics*, the *Guide for Professional Conduct*, and the *Standards of Physical Therapy Practice* (HOD 06-96-16-31)[12, 13] all include injunctions to provide informed consent. This obligation to provide informed consent is grounded in the principle of autonomy. Loewy[19] asserted that autonomy and beneficence are related in this case: "Caring enough for another's welfare to respect their autonomy, ultimately, is a beneficent thing to do." Although his observation may be true in a theoretical sense, it obscures the important distinction between obligations based on rights and obligations based on beneficence.

The *Guide for Professional Conduct* deals with informed consent under Principle 1 of *The Code of Ethics*. Principle 1 states that "Physical therapists respect the rights and dignity of all individuals."[13] Section 1.4 of the *Guide* states, "Physical therapists shall obtain patient informed consent before treatment, to include disclosure of: (i) the nature of the proposed intervention; (ii) material risks of harm or complications; (iii) reasonable alternatives to the proposed intervention; and (iv) goals of treatment." The *Standards of Practice for Physical Therapy and the Accompanying Criteria* elaborates this: "The physical therapist has sole responsibility for providing information to the patient/client and for obtaining the patient's/client's informed consent in accordance with jurisdictional law before initiating physical therapy."[12] This suggests that (1) obtaining informed consent is part of maintaining respect for the patient's rights (autonomy) and dignity, and (2) obtaining informed consent is a part of good physical therapy practice.

None of the relevant passages states that informed consent should be written. However, the APTA's standards continue to describe the initial evaluation, plan of care, treatment, and reevaluation. Under each of these subcategories, there is a specific statement that documentation should be provided. Should informed consent be written?

Undoubtedly most PTs believe that they obtain informed consent before beginning treatment. As professionals, PTs have prided themselves on the positive relationships that they have developed with patients during the rehabilitation process. A relationship of trust is a good foundation for obtaining informed consent. However, it may also contribute to patient exploitation. In the relationship between therapist and patient, there is a power imbalance because the therapist holds the relevant knowledge. Because patients trust and like their therapists, they may allow procedures to be performed that they do not truly understand.

For example, do patients really understand the risks and benefits of iontophoresis? Do therapists adequately disclose that there is a small risk that patients may sustain skin irritation or a small burn from the procedure? Of course it is impossible to disclose all information to each patient,[19] but do PTs have a process for providing the relevant information to each patient and ensuring that the patient understands and agrees?

As noted in the section *Informed Consent in the Research Setting*, a formalized process that produces written consent does not necessarily produce informed consent. Patients can easily sign what they do not read or understand. This is particularly true when obtaining informed consent is delegated to support personnel who do not themselves understand the procedures to which patients are consenting. However, the informal process of obtaining verbal consent to verbal disclosure is probably inadequate. On a busy day, are patients told that they can expect to be a little sore if they have not been exercising?

Is truly informed consent possible at all? In a study in which patients were interviewed regarding procedures they had consented to in writing the day before, only 60% understood the purpose and nature of the procedure, and only 55% correctly listed even one major risk or complication.[20] Three factors were related to inadequate recall: education, medical status, and the care with which patients thought they had read their consent forms before signing. Only 40% of the patients had read their consent carefully. Most believed that consent forms were meant to protect the physician's rights. Although most thought that consent forms were necessary and comprehensible and that they contained worthwhile information, the legalistic connotations of the forms appeared to lead to cursory reading and inadequate recall.

PTs (and other health care providers) may encounter institutional and economic obstacles to providing information to the patient as part of informed consent.[4] In some cases, managed care organizations have attempted to limit the information that providers give to patients. The purpose of gag clauses is presumably to decrease patient use of services. However, patients may be hesitant to trust business entities whose main purpose is to increase profits. (The problematic nature of business relationships in medicine is discussed in Chapter 3.)

The increasing trend to provide preventive care also presents challenges to informed consent.[21] Providing information about the possible ill effects of lifestyles requires far more time. What is adequate disclosure in this context? Are the long-term effects of certain lifestyles really known?

More specifically, to what extent are the risks and benefits of preventive screening programs known?[21] For example, many women older than 40 years began to have yearly mammograms in the belief that this was an effective measure against cancer. Evidence now suggests that mammograms are not effective in preventing cancer deaths until the age of 50 years. This situation illustrates the difficulty of disclosing and recommending when providers' own knowledge of the effectiveness of preventive measures is so small.

QUESTIONS AND NOTES FOR FURTHER REFLECTION

1. In a case involving a patient with spinal stenosis, a physician was found liable for improper treatment of the patient in the face of ongoing severe back pain.[22] Although the patient had not complained of pain to her physician, the physician was held to have knowledge of the complaints as documented by the PTs.

2. In your experience, how do PTs obtain informed consent? Should informed consent be obtained in writing?

3. Do PTs as professionals know the risks and benefits of the treatments provided? What kinds of studies can demonstrate the risks and benefits?

4. Have you experienced institutional barriers to providing disclosure to patients?

5. How does economic status (e.g., inability to pay, lack of insurance, small capitated rate) influence disclosure of therapeutic options?

6. For a discussion of these issues, see Purtilo[23] and Banja and Wolf.[24]

CASE 6.3

Kendra Links is a senior physical therapy student completing her final clinical affiliation in a private rehabilitation center. After evaluating a paraplegic patient who is human immunodeficiency virus (HIV) positive, Kendra asks her clinical supervisor whether the goals she has set for the patient are realistic. Her supervisor tells Kendra, "It does not really matter because we will refer him to General Hospital. We do not treat that kind of patient here.

After all, most of us have small children, you know." Kendra is stunned. What action should Kendra take?

LEGAL ANALYSIS: AMERICANS WITH DISABILITIES ACT COMPLIANCE

Legal Intervention

Title III of the Americans with Disabilities Act (ADA) (discussed in Chapter 4 with respect to employment issues) prohibits discrimination on the basis of disability in places of public accommodation. These include but are not limited to facilities such as schools, theaters, hospitals, hotels, and doctors' offices. Plaintiffs have been successful in bringing ADA lawsuits against physicians and dentists for refusing to treat them on the basis of a disability.[25, 26] In one case involving a dentist who refused to treat an HIV-positive individual, the plaintiff was awarded $25,000 for pain, humiliation, and emotional distress plus an additional $25,000 as punitive damages under the ADA. In addition to ADA and Rehabilitation Act claims, state human rights laws can also be added to the suit.

Hospitals have also been subject to litigation under the ADA. In *Howe v. Hull*,[27] an individual presented to the emergency room with an acute severe allergic reaction to a new prescription medication. The physician refused to admit the patient because the patient was HIV positive, despite the fact that the acute condition was unrelated to his seropositive status. The patient successfully brought suit against the physician and the facility. Another case involved a deaf woman who was unable to communicate with hospital staff during her husband's admission.[28] The hospital failed to show ADA compliance or that hiring an interpreter would have posed an undue burden. Refusal to treat an acquired immune deficiency syndrome (AIDS) patient provided sufficient grounds for termination of a pregnant home health nurse and did not constitute a violation of the Pregnancy Discrimination Act.[29]

Despite these cases, however, physicians (and presumably other health care professionals) can refer patients to other health care providers on the basis of the disability if the individual requires treatment or services outside the referring provider's area of specialization.[30] Thus, it would be permissible for a speech pathologist to refer a deaf individual who had suffered a stroke to another speech pathologist who knows sign language.

Application to Case 6.3

Kendra's clinical instructor appears to be impermissibly discriminating against the patient on the basis of his disability. Absent a reason to refer (e.g., General Hospital has a superior spinal cord unit), liability may be imposed under the ADA. Kendra is not under a legal obligation, however, to report her supervisor.

ETHICAL ANALYSIS

Case 6.3 raises the question of professionals' obligation to treat, as well as the issue of justice. It was noted in the discussion of professions in Chapter 2 that society has granted professionals a great deal of autonomy in exchange for self-regulation. Some ethicists describe this as a kind of social contract. As Loewy[19] described it, "A view of what we owe to one another as individuals, as professionals, and as members of the community when faced with a fear of 'coming to harm' is inevitably grounded in our view of social contract: both the wider understandings of our society and the more specific understandings of our professional group or institution." A social contract view would imply that the autonomy granted to professionals comes with the obligation to exercise responsibility.

Although the *Code* and *Guide* offer no explicit references to treating individuals with infectious diseases, an obligation not to discriminate against persons with AIDS is implicit in 1.1B of the *Guide*: "Physical therapists are to be guided at all times by concern for the physical, psychological, and socioeconomic welfare of those individuals entrusted to their care."[13]

The APTA House of Delegates issued a position on infectious diseases in 1989 (HOD 06-89-39-84):

> Physical therapy practitioners have an obligation to provide quality, nonjudgmental care in accordance with their knowledge and expertise to all persons who need it, regardless of the nature of the health problem. When providing care to individuals, the Association advocates that members be guided in their actions by guidelines developed by the Centers for Disease Control and Prevention (CDC) and regulations set by the Occupational Safety and Health Administration (OSHA).

Similarly, the House of Delegate's statement titled *Physical Therapy Services: Access, Admission and Patients' Rights* (HOD 06-93-16-22) states, "In providing physical therapy services, the physical therapist is accountable first and foremost to the individual receiving physical therapy.... The physical therapist shall ensure services regardless of race, creed, color, gender, age, national or ethnic origin, sexual orientation, disability or health status."

These and other statements make it clear that Kendra's clinical instructor has a responsibility to treat patients who are HIV positive.

At the same time, she should use the infection control measures outlined by the CDC and OSHA.

Questions for Further Reflection

1. How should PTs and physical therapist assistants deal with the fear that is associated with AIDS?

2. What other obligations to society are inherent in being a PT?

3. In the past, epidemics have afflicted most societies. Before modern ability to contain communication of disease, physicians and nurses had to decide whether they should expose themselves to the risk of contracting a disease. What obligation, if any, do PTs have to treat a disease that could not be contained? How would you approach such a decision?

CASE 6.4

Richard Rodriguez is the academic clinical coordinator in the physical therapy program at East Bay University. On Monday morning, he receives a phone call from Mary Beckley, who is a junior student placed at Bayview Physical Therapy, a private practice. Mary tells him that she is considering accepting a position with Bayview after graduation. Bayview has asked Mary to sign a 3-year, noncompete contract. In exchange for employment, Bayview will pay for Mary's senior year of education. This contract stipulates that she cannot accept employment at any other facility within 50 miles of Bayview within 3 years of terminating employment at Bayview. Mary has very few financial resources. She is a single mother and badly needs money for the next year of school. She has called Richard to request advice about whether to sign this agreement.

LEGAL ANALYSIS: NONCOMPETE CLAUSES

Noncompete clauses, also referred to as covenants not to compete, must be reasonable in scope, duration, and geographic area and must relate to a legally protectible interest of the employer to be enforceable. In addition, there must be something of value given in exchange for the agreement. When an employee is serving at will and can thus be fired at any time, some courts have held that there is insufficient consideration to support a noncompete clause.

What constitutes reasonable duration and geographic scope? This determination is largely dependent on the situation and requires a case-by-case analysis. The matter is governed by state law. Some states have laws addressing such covenants, giving specific time limits. Louisiana law, for example, provides that such clauses are not to exceed a period of 2 years.[31] Others are more general in nature. Wisconsin law, for example, requires that the covenant (1) be necessary to protect the employer, (2) provide reasonable time restrictions, (3) provide a reasonable territorial limit, (4) must not be harsh or oppressive to the employee, and (5) must not be contrary to public policy.[32] These principles reflect the general common law regarding covenants not to compete and have been applied in several medical cases as discussed in the following section.

A physical therapy noncompete clause was struck down in *Concept Rehab Inc. v. Short.*[33] The contract imposed a 2-year noncompete clause extending to "any patient of any customer of the corporation." The appeals court found that to uphold the clause would create an undue hardship on the therapist and impose an absurd requirement that she do a detailed background check on any patient transferred into her care.

In a case involving a speech therapist, a 2-year covenant not to compete was struck down by a Louisiana court as void for failing to explicitly define the employer's business.[34] The court documents described the agency as "a certified rehabilitation agency providing therapy services in the field of speech pathology, vocational rehabilitation, occupational therapy, physical therapy, and social work services." Such language was not contained in the agreement, however, and was arguably too broad to withstand scrutiny under Louisiana law, which does not favor restrictive covenants.

In physician cases, covenants to compete have been invalidated as against public policy when a physician serves as the only specialist within a region.[35] Other covenants have been modified for public policy considerations. Thus, in a covenant specifying that an orthopedic surgeon could not practice at a clinic or hospital within a 5-mile radius of the clinics of his former employer, the court modified the agreement to permit the surgeon to treat his patients presenting to an emergency room within the 5-mile zone.[36] The agreement, which was for a period of 2 years, was otherwise held enforceable. In a Wisconsin case involving a physician employed by a pain clinic, the court upheld a restrictive covenant for a period of 1 year within a 20-mile radius; the physician was also prohibited from soliciting former patients of the pain center for a period of 2 years.[37]

In considering the reasonableness of geographic scope, courts appraise the business of the employer and its market. Duration should reflect a reasonable need of the employer while not imposing an undue hardship on the former employee.[38]

Application to Case 6.4

Outcomes in restrictive covenant cases are very difficult to predict as they are quite fact specific and dependent on state law. There does appear to be consideration for the agreement, both through employment and payment, for Mary's senior year of school. In assessing the covenant, the court will look to the reasonableness of the restriction: Does it pose an undue hardship on the employee? Is it a reasonable protection of the employer's interest? Does the clinic's patient base extend to a 50-mile radius? Is the duration reasonable? Presuming Mary brings no particular clinical expertise to the area, the contract would likely not be void on public policy grounds.

ETHICAL ANALYSIS

The ethical concern in Case 6.4 relates to the undue influence that financial considerations play in the student's determination of professional choices. The additional concern is that students, who do not yet have experience, may enter into an agreement the ramifications and consequences of which they may not truly understand. In effect, students may be trading their professional future for the present. Many times the contract has unforeseen consequences: Ownership may change or staffing changes may result in the student's being sent to a facility other than the one originally discussed. Although there is nothing intrinsically unethical about offering or accepting a contract for future employment, there is a concern that students may not be negotiating as equals with respect to employers.

To assist students and schools who advise students, the APTA's House of Delegates in 1992 established *Guidelines for Student and Employer Contracts* (HOD 06-92-14-28):

1. Notification by the employer if the place of employment may be in an isolated area or as a solo practitioner such that the new graduate will not have ready access to mentoring and regular collegial relationships or any resources for professional growth and development.
2. Disclosure by the employer of ownership of the practice.

3. Notification by the employer to the student if the practice is involved in any situation in which a referring practitioner can profit as a result of referring patients for physical therapy and notification that the American Physical Therapy Association (APTA) is opposed to such situations.
4. Student awareness of any potential future tax obligations that may be incurred upon graduation as the result of deferred income.
5. The agreement must not, in any way, interfere with the process and planning of the student's professional education.
6. It should be understood that the school is not a party to the agreement and is not bound to any conditions of the agreement.
7. There should be a clearly delineated, fair and reasonable buy out provision in which the student understands the legal commitment to pay back the stipend with reasonable interest in the event that there is dissatisfaction or reason for release from the contract on the student's part at any time during the term of the agreement.
8. A no penalty bailout provision should be provided in the event of change of ownership, but the student may be required to adhere to a reasonable payback schedule.
9. Avoidance of non-compete clauses is recommended but if there is one, a reasonable limitation of time and distance should be incorporated.
10. A student's interests may be best served by obtaining appropriate counsel before signing the contract.

During the recent past, the shortage of PTs resulted in a number of students entering into employer contracts. Many students subsequently accepted positions with other employers who were willing to buy out the original contract from the initial employer. Employers were, in essence, in a bidding war for the services of new graduates.

QUESTIONS FOR FURTHER REFLECTION

1. How should one view contracts with future employers? Is a contract for future employment like a commodity that can be sold, or does it represent a personal commitment to act in good faith?

2. Are the APTA House of Delegate guidelines adequate to protect the interests of all parties involved: students, employers, the school, and the profession? What other guidelines would you suggest?

3. Why do the guidelines discourage new PTs from accepting employment in solo practices or remote areas?

4. What are the consequences for the profession, for medical practice, and for the general public of the personnel shortage in physical therapy? What will happen to the profession when the personnel shortage ends?

CASE 6.5

Maggie Overbrook and Dean Huddington are students at the Oak
Valley University Physical Therapy Department. They are assigned
to complete their final clinical education component at Green-
wood Physical Therapy Clinic. On the first morning of the rotation, they meet with the clinic owner, Gwen Strickland, PT, for
orientation to the rotation. After reviewing policies and procedures, Gwen describes the clientele of the clinic. Many of the
patients are women with pelvic pain and incontinence. She hands
Maggie and Dean a packet of copyrighted protocols that describe
the treatment progression for pelvic pain, postpartum recovery,
and incontinence due to pelvic floor dysfunction. Some of the
protocols call for precise parameters using a specialized electrical
stimulator. The three of them discuss the sequences of treatment,
and Gwen answers their questions. At the end of their meeting,
the students put the materials into their notebooks. Gwen stops
them to ask for the protocols back, saying, "I really cannot let you
have a copy of those protocols. It has taken me 10 years to
develop a specialty referral base. Right now, I am the only PT in
the valley who provides this type of service. Next year, one of you
might take a job at Oak Valley Hospital and use my protocols to
compete with me." Dean and Maggie wonder how they will be
able to carry out the treatment without having the written protocols available. Gwen assures them that she will assist them
whenever needed.

LEGAL ANALYSIS: INTELLECTUAL PROPERTY

The conduct as described is legally permissible; facilities are within
their rights to withhold such materials. However, liability may attach
if a patient is injured by a negligent student inadequately supervised
and unfamiliar with the proper protocol. Furthermore, the case illustrates the tension between law and ethics in an increasingly corporate
health care environment. Legally, the protection of ideas (known as
intellectual property) has typically been undertaken through patent
and copyright laws. Patent law, established under Article 1, Section 8,
of the U.S. Constitution, states, "The Congress shall have the power
... to promote the progress of science and useful arts, by securing for
limited times to authors and inventors the exclusive right to their
respective writings and discoveries." If an unauthorized person uses a
patented invention or process, that individual may be subject to liability for patent infringement. This is true even if the person acted

without knowledge of the patent. Patents have been issued for medical procedures, including a patent for a stitch-free incision for the removal of cataracts. The patent holder sued another physician for patent infringement.[39]

The inherent tension between protection of intellectual property rights and the need to disseminate medical knowledge led to modifications to federal patent law that limit patent infringement suits relating to a medical practitioner's performance of a medical activity.[40] The law provides that health care practitioners cannot enforce patents for medical procedures against other providers or hospitals. The law does not apply to patents issued before its enactment.

In discussions about the proposed legislation, supporters of the bill, including the American Medical Association (AMA), argued that patents have no place in medicine due to the need to disseminate information. The AMA issued a statement that it is "unethical for physicians to seek, secure, or enforce patents on medical procedures."[41] Critics, including the Patent and Technology Office and the American Bar Association, believe that elimination of patent protection will diminish research funding.

ETHICAL ANALYSIS

Case 6.5 presents important concerns about the nature of professional relationships, responsibilities to future colleagues, and responsibility to society. The nature of professions was discussed in Chapter 2. Professional societies are assumed to regulate the education of their members. The introduction of the business perspective to health care has created a shift in attitude, however; Gwen views students as future competitors rather than as future colleagues. This is an important shift in perspective and in relationship.

Most professional codes bid health care providers to place the interests of patients and society ahead of their own interests. It would be difficult to argue the permissibility of patents from the standpoint of beneficence or justice. (Patents restrict access to state-of-the-art medical treatment.) However, it can be argued that, viewing justice as merit, one ought to be able to reap the benefits of one's effort.

QUESTIONS FOR FURTHER REFLECTION

1. Do professional obligations include education of future colleagues?

2. How should self-interest be balanced with the needs for society in a business-dominated medical environment?

3. From a business perspective, medical knowledge and health care are commodities. What are the ramifications of this view for physical therapy?

4. The Family Education Rights and Privacy Act (FERPA) provides protection of privacy for educational records, with some exceptions.[42] There are exceptions for so-called directory data and for information release to parents that declare the student as a dependent on federal income tax forms. Federal funding is made conditional on compliance with FERPA. Can you think of legal and ethical issues that might be associated with FERPA?

CASE FOR FURTHER REFLECTION

Michelle Harrison is a PT at Mercy Hospital, a suburban hospital in a Midwestern town. Michelle is the only PT at Mercy who is African American. During her 20 years of physical therapy practice, she has become increasingly concerned about the small percentage of PTs who are members of a minority group. Michelle has attempted to improve this situation by speaking to high school and church groups, by serving on the admissions committee of the local physical therapy program, and by mentoring students on their clinical rotation at Mercy. Michelle remembers how lonely it was to be the only African-American student in her physical therapy class.

There are currently two students completing their rotations at Mercy. Mercy uses a 2 to 1 student-to-instructor model. Craig Raskin serves as clinical instructor to both students: Dan Villet and Shawna Daniels. Shawna is one of three African-American students in her class. Although Shawna did well in her previous affiliations, she has struggled throughout this affiliation. Michelle supervised Shawna for 2 days while Craig was ill and thought that Shawna was above average in both clinical skills and knowledge base.

A week before the final day of the affiliation, Shawna enters Michelle's office very upset. Craig has just informed her that he will probably be unable to pass her for the affiliation. This came as a total surprise to Shawna. Shawna tells Michelle that Craig is more critical of her work because she is African American. On one occasion, Shawna overheard Craig sharing a racist joke with another employee. Shawna asks Michelle to intervene on her behalf.

Michelle thinks that this is a difficult situation. She has never taken a high-profile stance against discrimination. She does not like racial controversy. Their staff is very small, and Craig is well liked by everyone; Michelle has concerns about opposing him. At the same time, Michelle sees some basis for Shawna's complaints. In 5 years of clinical supervision, Craig has rarely had doubts about passing white students, but he has failed three African-American students. Craig once commented to Michelle that African-American students seemed less prepared for affiliations than other students. Michelle wonders what she should do. A part of her feels that it is time to stand up to an unfair system, but she does not want to lose the good working relationships she has worked so hard to cultivate. What is the right thing to do, she wonders.

QUESTIONS FOR FURTHER REFLECTION

1. What ethical and legal issues does this case raise?

2. In spite of the numerous policies and positions of the APTA regarding affirmative action and nondiscrimination, the profession continues to experience difficulty recruiting minorities. In fact, fewer than 6% of PTs are minorities.[43] Why is this? What effect does this have on the profession?

3. A journal article reported the results of a study comparing grading of minority students and white students.[43] Students were given identical reports to present. African-American and other minority students were given lower grades for the same presentation. How should biases, known and unknown, in educational judgments be handled? What are the ramifications for health care delivery of "covert bias"?[43]

REFERENCES

1. U.S. Department of Health and Human Services Policy for Protection of Human Research Subjects, 45 C.F.R. §46, 101.
2. Katz J. Informed Consent in the Therapeutic Relationship: Law and Ethics. In WT Reich (ed), Encyclopedia of Bioethics (Vol 2). New York: Free Press, 1978;770, 771.
3. Beauchamp TL, Childress JF. Principles of Biomedical Ethics (4th ed). New York: Oxford University Press, 1994;142, 145–147.
4. Levinsky NG. Social, institutional, and economic barriers to the exercise of patients' rights. N Engl J Med 1996;334:532.
5. Annas GJ, Grodin MA (eds). The Nazi Doctors and the Nuremberg Code: Human Rights in Human Experimentation. New York: Oxford University Press, 1992;3.

6. Perley S, Fluss SS, Bankowski Z, Simon F. The Nuremberg Code: An International Overview. In GJ Annas, MA Grodin (eds), The Nazi Doctors and the Nuremberg Code: Human Rights in Human Experimentation. New York: Oxford University Press, 1992;149–173.
7. Advisory Committee on Human Radiation Experimentation. Report of the Advisory Committee on Human Radiation Experimentation. Washington, DC: Government Printing Office, 1995.
8. Katz J. Statement by Individual Committee Member. In Report of the Advisory Committee on Human Radiation Experimentation. Washington, DC: Government Printing Office, 1995.
9. Purtilo R. Ethical Dimensions in the Health Professions (2nd ed). Philadelphia: Saunders, 1993;39.
10. Smith H. Introduction to legal risks associated with clinical education. J Phys Ther Ed 1994;8:67.
11. Scott R. CIs and liability. PT Mag 1995;3:30.
12. American Physical Therapy Association. Standards of Practice for Physical Therapy and the Accompanying Criteria. Alexandria, VA: American Physical Therapy Association, 1996.
13. American Physical Therapy Association. Guide for Professional Conduct. Alexandria, VA: American Physical Therapy Association. 1997.
14. *Canterbury v. Spence*, 464 F.2d 772 (D.C. Cir. 1972); *cert. denied*, 409 U.S. 1064 (1972).
15. Scott R. Forum on ethics: informed consent. Presented at the CPA-APTA Joint Congress; 1994; Toronto, Canada.
16. Scott R. Legal Aspects of Documenting Patient Care. Gaithersburg, MD: Aspen, 1994.
17. *Dorko v. Ohio Occupational Therapy* (Ohio App. Summit Co. 1992) 8 A.L.R. 5th 825.
18. *Enaw v. Dowling* 72657 (N.Y. App. Div. Oct. 26, 1995).
19. Loewy EH. Textbook of Healthcare Ethics. New York: Plenum, 1996;115, 119, 133.
20. Cassileth B, Zupkis R, Sutton-Smith K, March V. Informed consent—why are its goals imperfectly realized? N Engl J Med 1980;302:896.
21. Marshall KG. Prevention: how much harm? How much benefit? 4. The ethics of informed consent for preventive screening programs. J Can Med Assoc 1996;155:377.
22. *Bilderback v. Priestley*, 709 S.W.2d 736 (Tex. App. San Antonio 1986).
23. Purtilo R. Applying ethical principles of informed consent to patient care. Phys Ther 1994;64:934–937.
24. Banja J, Wolf S. Malpractice litigation for uninformed consent. Phys Ther 1982;67:1226–1229.
25. *D.B. v. Bloom*, 896 F. Supp. 166 (D.N.J. 1995).
26. *U.S. v. Morvant*, 898 F. Supp. 157 (1995).
27. *Howe v. Hull*, 874 F. Supp. 779 (1994).
28. *Aikens v. St. Helena Hosp.*, 843 F. Supp. 1329 (N.D.Cal. 1994).
29. *Armstrong v. Flowers Hospital*, 33 F.3d 1308 (11th Cir. 1994).
30. Modifications in Policies, Practices, or Procedures. 28 C.F.R. §36.302(b)(2).
31. Louisiana Revised Statutes ch 23, §921 (c).
32. Wisconsin Statutes Annotated ch 103, §465 (West 1988).

33. *Concept Rehab Inc. v. Short*, F-96-019 (Fulton County Ct. of App.); 95CV000121 (March 7, 1997).
34. *LaFourche Speech & Language Services, Inc v. Juckett*, 652 So.2d 679 (La. App. 1st Cir. 1995).
35. *Hoddeson v. Conroe Ear, Nose & Throat Assocs., P.C.*, 751 S.W.2d 289 (Tex. Ct. App. 1988).
36. *Phoenix Orthopaedic Surgeons v. Peairs*, 790 P.2d 752 (Ariz. App. 1989).
37. *Pollack v. Calimag*, 458 N.W.2d 591, 157 Wis.2d 222 (1990).
38. Decker K. Covenants Not to Compete (2nd ed). New York: Wiley, 1993.
39. *Samuel Pallin, M.D. v. Jack Singer, M.D. and the Hitchcock Clinic*, 1995 WL 608365 (D.Vt. May 1, 1995).
40. Limitations on Patent Infringements Relating to a Medical Practitioner's Performance of a Medical Activity, 35 U.S.C.A. §287(c)(1).
41. Report 1 of the Council on Ethical and Judicial Affairs (A-95), Patenting of Medical Procedures.
42. 20 U.S.C.A. §1232(g).
43. Haskins AR, Rose-St Prix C, Elbaum L. Covert bias in evaluation of PT students' clinical performance. Phys Ther 1997;77:155–168.

7

Emerging and Future Ethical and Legal Issues in Physical Therapy

Traditionally, the quality and effectiveness of health care have been assessed by using the concepts of quality, cost, and access. Presumably, the best health care delivery system represents a perfect balance between the three (Figure 7.1). In addition, each historical period tends to emphasize a different principle. Concerns about access of elderly and poor persons to health care during the 1950s and 1960s brought about the passage of Medicare and Medicaid during the 1960s. Widespread availability of health insurance during the 1970s allowed the health care delivery system to concentrate on issues of quality, including technological advances. For multiple reasons, medical care ultimately became too costly during the 1980s and 1990s. Accordingly, concerns of quality gave way to concerns of cost. Although President Bill Clinton's defeated health care proposal emphasized access, efforts since that time have continued to focus on cost.[1] Some would argue that cost-containment is emphasized at the expense of both quality and access (Figure 7.2).

This chapter discusses resources to deal with legal and ethical matters, litigation preparation, alternative dispute solution, influencing legislation, and future issues, areas in which legal or ethical issues, or both, may arise.

The focus of health care delivery at any given time impacts on both ethical and legal debates. For example, when the emphasis of health care during the 1960s and 1970s was on access and quality, ethical debate centered largely on autonomy, patients' rights, and informed consent. Legal debate brought these same issues to the courts, asking for financial awards when these principles were abrogated. In the current managed care age, as the system focuses on cost-containment, there is a simultaneous reaction that raises issues of access and quality to the fore. For example, managed care systems are being asked to pro-

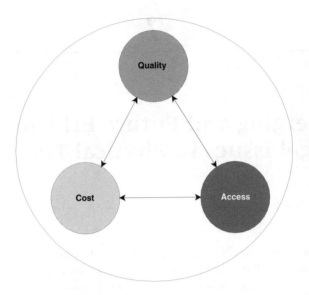

Figure 7.1 Focus of ideal health care delivery system with balance between elements.

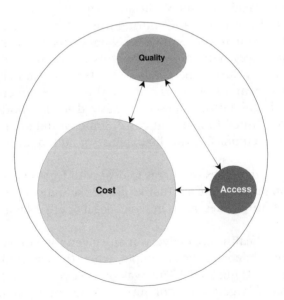

Figure 7.2 Health care delivery system focused on cost at the expense of access and quality. Demonstrates an imbalance between elements.

vide systems of due process to adjudicate disputes about appropriate treatment. This debate suggests that the paradigm shift toward a business perspective in managed care is not yet complete. The new paradigm of health care delivery will not likely be a system so shifted toward cost, but may be more balanced between the three traditional elements: quality, cost, and access.

The focus of the health care delivery system is shaped by multiple social, political, and personal forces, as well as by multiple actors. (See Chapter 1 and Figures 1.1–1.3 for a review of the web of relationships in which health care occurs.) Legislative action, judicial decision, professional association standards, and corporate practices are currently playing an important role in shaping the focus of health care delivery. The push to focus primarily on cost of health care seems to be shifting toward a more balanced approach.

Ethical quandaries are inherent to the delivery of health care. The quality and length of people's lives are at stake. The development in the United States of the third-party-payer, fee-for-service system has increased the number and complexity of ethical problems encountered. Rapid technological advances in the 1970s created unique ethical dilemmas that traditional approaches were unable to solve.

PHILOSOPHICAL PRINCIPLES

Since its beginnings in the 1970s, medical ethics has relied on philosophical principles. The principles of autonomy, beneficence, nonmaleficence, and justice have provided valuable tools for clinicians to approach the problems inherent in delivering medical care. Increasing emphasis on patients' rights, acknowledgment of inherent gender perspectives, disillusionment with the hierarchical structure of medicine, inequities in resource allocation, and conflicting principles have all pointed to the shortcomings of the principle-based approach. In addition, the principles approach has proved inadequate in suggesting viable social and systemic reforms of the health care system.

Feminist critics, the ethics of care, contextualism, and casuistry all present important alternatives to the four principles approach. However, these perspectives represent a valuable adjunct to the principles approach rather than a substitute for it. The four principles approach is now the official language and tradition of medical ethics. It provides the terms by which dilemmas are conceptualized and the bridge by which past conversations are linked with the present. Its language has shaped the codes of ethics of most medical professional groups, including those in physical therapy. Beyond that, the principles capture fundamental ethical norms. Although other perspectives may correct for the deficiencies of the principle approach, it is unlikely that it will be supplanted in the near future. The four principles will continue to play a major role in medical ethics and in ethics for physical therapists (PTs) and physical therapist assistants (PTAs).

BUSINESS PERSPECTIVES

Rapid changes in the 1990s and the shift of medicine toward business perspectives will continue to pose challenges for traditional approaches. Resolving ethical issues related to access and justice, never the strong point of the traditional approach, will be even more problematic when approached from the perspective of business ethics. The increasing business perspective of medicine will force the medical professions to look more carefully at their roles and responsibilities. Although business interests will push increasingly for the deprofessionalization of medicine in the interest of decreasing costs, physical therapy must evaluate its rights and responsibilities in the health care system.

Accountability

Corporatization of medical care will also increase calls for accountability. In some cases, as is currently happening, accountability will come through judicial review. Legislation will undoubtedly address additional concerns about accountability. PTs and other health care providers will be more accountable for their use of health care dollars. If the predominant ethical dilemma of the last few decades has been balancing autonomy and beneficence, the dilemma of the next decade may be balancing accountability and justice in allocation. Conflict of interest will continue to be a focus of ethical debate.

Reliability

An underlying issue for physical therapy is the availability of reliable outcomes data. Accountability to the system will demand valid and reliable data on which to base decisions. When PTs recommend a particular course of treatment, the expectation will be that the potential outcome and cost of such a treatment is known. Similarly, the expectation will be that as a profession PTs have reached some agreement on the optimal approach to a particular patient's problems.

Patients' Rights

Since the late 1970s, there has been a remarkable growth in advocacy for patients' rights. How will these rights be protected in corporate medicine? PTs will increasingly be called on to advocate for patients and to play a role in ensuring protection of patients' rights.

LEGAL AND ETHICAL MATTERS IN THE CLINICAL SETTING

If a legal or ethical matter presents itself in the clinical setting, to whom should PTs turn first? Of course, this is necessarily a fact-based analysis. However, as indicated in Chapter 1, turning to colleagues and professional resources (such as the American Physical Therapy Association's [APTA] *Guide for Professional Conduct*) helps to define whether a dilemma is a legal matter, an ethical matter, both, or neither. Any information shared with colleagues in consultation about such issues must protect the confidentiality of the people involved.

If the situation occurs in a hospital environment, there are typically additional resources to consult. In addition to reporting or discussing matters of concern with supervisory staff, and depending on the nature of the problem, one might consider consultation with the house ethics committee. Ethics committees are interdisciplinary committees that consider issues of patient rights; their recommendations are usually advisory in situations in which patient or family wishes conflict with those of a treating physician. (See Chapter 5 for a discussion of ethics committees.)

In-house counsel refers to the attorneys who represent the hospital. Such attorneys are employed directly by the hospital; some facilities use attorneys associated with law firms for all their legal work. Most hospitals use law firm attorneys for litigation needs. If a legal problem arises, it may be advisable to consult with the hospital attorney. However, should the therapist have a concern regarding conflicting interests vis-à-vis those of the hospital, it is advisable to seek independent counsel for advice. When consulting with an attorney, it is important to disclose all known facts and sources of information and to be completely truthful. Such discussions are generally protected under attorney-client privilege.

If a potential legal or ethical problem arises, the hospital risk-management department should also be made aware of the situation. (See Chapter 4 for a discussion of risk-management principles.) Some situations warrant being reported to the state licensure board or to the ethics committee of the state chapter of the APTA.

LITIGATION

This section discusses the phases of litigation and some general tips about preparation for involvement in the process, including depositions.

Process

The first step in the litigation process involves filing a complaint. The plaintiff must file the lawsuit in a timely manner—that is, within the statute of limitations for the particular action. This time frame is established by state or federal law and is specific to the type of suit. For example, state statutes of limitation for medical malpractice cases are generally from 1 to 3 years, with some exceptions for minors and in cases involving fraudulent concealment. If the plaintiff fails to bring the case within the required time limit, the suit is dismissed.

Once a complaint is filed, a summons, or service, is issued to inform the defendant(s) about the case. Defendants should make their insurance representatives aware of such summons immediately, as some policies make prompt notification a prerequisite of coverage. Pleadings are then submitted to the court; these provide each party's version of the facts of the case and the legal basis for the claim. Defendants submit an answer that may include counterclaims. If the pleadings involve only issues of law and if there is no factual dispute, the judge may decide the matter through a motion based on the pleadings alone. Otherwise, a trial is needed to clarify factual inconsistencies.

In preparing for trial, the attorneys issue interrogatories (written questions about the case) for response by the opposing party. They also take depositions (oral responses to questions); these responses are recorded by a court reporter and may be referenced during the trial. In responding to questions, either through depositions or interrogatories (or when a witness at trial), it is important to be brief. Witnesses should answer only the question posed, not volunteer extraneous information, take their time and ask for clarification, if necessary, and be absolutely honest, as they are under oath. When testifying about something about which a witness does not have independent knowledge (that he or she has read about or that someone else has stated), the source of the information must be disclosed. Preparation is essential, including discussion with the attorney. The opposing attorney is in the position of vigorously advocating for the client. He or she will tend to emphasize the strengths of his or her party's case and may attempt to have the deponent give contradictory statements, at times bullying or ridiculing. (Witnesses should not be misled, however, by an overly friendly opposing attorney who asks seemingly casual, offhand questions; this may be another technique to extract information.)

Preparation

Therapists deposed as fact witnesses, rather than as a party to the case, should not assume that preparation is unnecessary. If involved in the case in any way, the therapist may later be added as a defendant based on statements made in the deposition. Therapists who provide expert witness testimony should also prepare fully for depositions, whether asked to testify regarding the extent of injury, the standard of care, or both. Objectivity is critical. As stated by Brimer,[2] a potential expert witness must be able to answer four questions before agreeing to serve as an expert.

1. Am I qualified to testify as to the proper standards of care in this instance?
2. If so, did the care given by the therapist in this case meet those standards?
3. If it failed to do so, could I testify that injury may have ensued as a result of negligence on the part of the therapist?
4. Can I present the issue as clear-cut and easy for lay people to understand, so that the case will be easy to present or even settle out of court?

Settlement

A number of issues may be dealt with at pretrial hearings, in court, or at more informal pretrial conferences. Unless the matter is settled, it then proceeds to trial. A jury is selected, both attorneys offer opening statements, and the plaintiff's attorney begins the case by calling witnesses. As in deposition, information is presented through a question-and-answer format, and the recommendations regarding deposition testimony also apply at trial. Following presentation of the plaintiff's witness, the defense attorney has an opportunity for cross-examination. The plaintiff's attorney can then ask additional questions of the witnesses to try to overcome statements made during cross-examination. At the close of the plaintiff's case, the defense attorney can move for a directed verdict (a statement by the judge that the plaintiff has failed to state a case and that the matter should be dismissed). If the motion is denied, the defendant's case is presented. Motions may be made that the defense or the complaint were inadequate. If overruled, the judge then instructs the jury as to the applicable law and the jury deliberates to reach a verdict. After the verdict is rendered, the losing party may request a new trial. If denied, the matter is final, subject to appeal.

ALTERNATIVE DISPUTE RESOLUTION

Another method of dispute determination is known as *alternative dispute resolution*, which refers to mediation, arbitration, or some other form of dispute resolution to which the parties agree. Arbitration is the submission of a dispute for settlement to a third person or to a panel of experts outside the judicial trial process.[3] In contrast, mediation involves a third party, who attempts to assist the parties in reaching a settlement; mediation is typically not binding. These forums are agreed to in advance (e.g., in a contract for services or at the time a dispute arises) or are mandated by statute. Alternative dispute resolution offers some advantages in terms of cost and speed over traditional litigation. In addition, panel members may have expertise in a particular area of controversy, as opposed to judges, who are generally experts only in the legal elements posed by a case. Health care professionals may also find themselves more comfortable in an environment that is somewhat less confrontational and adversarial than traditional legal proceedings. Such tribunals do not establish precedent for other cases but apply only to the parties engaged in a dispute.

INFLUENCING LEGISLATION

With numerous changes on the horizon in the delivery of and payment for health care services and with increasing autonomy and responsibility, PTs as professionals must be aware of means of influencing legislation on both federal and state levels. PTs may stay current on pending legislation via the Internet. One means of influencing legislatures is through political action committee (PAC) contributions. APTA staff members also advocate on behalf of the interests of the members. For example, the APTA ran an advertisement in *The Washington Post* and *Roll Call* captioned, "To Remind Congress of the Cost-Saving Benefits of Physical Therapy on Total U.S. Health Care Spending, We Thought We'd Send Them a Card." The card depicted read, "Get Well Sooner!" and was sent to each of the U.S. senators and representatives. The *PTeam Alert*, by the APTA's Grassroots Network, updates members about pending and recent legislation.

Several APTA chapters have sponsored creative efforts, including health and fitness screenings, to become acquainted with state legislators and to educate them about physical therapy.[4] Many chapters employ lobbyists or have volunteer legislative liaisons to keep track of legislation with a potential impact on physical therapy. Collaboration with other professional associations in areas of mutual interest is also helpful. Direct written communications and personal visits with both state and federal legislators remain important.[5] Physical therapy educators may make tracking and acting on proposed legislation a student assignment.

FUTURE TRENDS

This section addresses future trends and areas that may be a source of legal and ethical issues, including multi-skilling, telemedicine, insurance mandates, access to care, and future trends in ethical analysis.

Multi-Skilling

Multi-skilling, or cross-training, is an issue that is receiving considerable attention in health care. As a legal matter, a PT should not be called on to render services that fall outside the definition of physical therapy contained in the state practice act. Neither should unqualified individuals be asked to provide physical therapy care. The position of the APTA House of Delegates with respect to multi-skilling is as follows:

> The American Physical Therapy Association (APTA) opposes the concept of the multi-skilled professional practitioner, defined as "a health care practitioner who is cross-trained in area(s) of practice in which the individual is neither educated nor licensed." The APTA opposes cross-training of physical therapists and physical therapist assistants in areas outside the scope of physical therapy practice. The APTA also opposes cross-training of other health care practitioners into physical therapy practice. This position should not be interpreted as expressing opposition to coordination of care involving professional practitioners from different disciplines or dual-credentialing through education and licensure.
>
> The APTA supports the utilization of multi-skilled (cross-trained) support personnel who perform delegated components of physical therapy intervention under the direct supervision of physical therapists and physical therapist assistants in accordance with state laws and regulations. Multi-skilled support personnel refers to individuals with "on-the-job training within applicable state laws and regulations to provide services outside or in addition to the scope of their educational preparation or training." When multi-skilled (cross-trained) personnel perform delegated tasks other than those delegated under the direction of a physical therapist, they should be under the direct supervision of an appropriate licensed health practitioner (HOD 06-95-27-17).

Telemedicine

The advent of telemedicine also raises interesting and unanswered liability issues. Several courts have refused to impose liability for physicians consulting via the telephone. For example, in a Texas case, no liability was imposed on a physician consulted by telephone by an emergency room physician.[6] These cases generally are grounded in the theory that no physician-patient relationship exists. However, the result would likely be different in cases in which the relationship is clearly established.

The Health Insurance Portability and Accountability Act of 1996 provides for a study to be performed by the Health Care Financing Administration for submission to Congress about telemedicine.[7] A report from the Physician Insurers Association of America (PIAA), *Telemedicine: An Overview of Applications and Barriers*, stated that legal issues are the biggest barrier to growth of telemedicine.[8, 9] The report suggested that because the referring physician retains the choice as to whether to act on the consultant's advice, "it could be argued that the referring physician vicariously assumes all risk for the acts of the teleconsultant." Issues of confidentiality may be particularly problematic with some forms of modern telecommunication.

Insurance Mandates

Another area of possible action is in insurance mandates. These are legislatively created requirements to provide care. As discussed in Chapter 3, some states have adopted such mandates with respect to managed care organizations (MCOs). Another example is the creation of a specific federal statute that mandates insurance coverage of 48-hour hospital stays for new mothers and infants following delivery.[10] The public and legislators perceive insurance company determinations to encroach on traditional determinations of medical necessity by health care providers, and as providers PTs can anticipate additional impetus toward such mandates. The APTA has endorsed the Women's Health and Cancer Rights Act, which mandates coverage of second opinions for breast, colon, and prostate cancer diagnoses. The legislation also guarantees 48 hours of inpatient care following a mastectomy and 24 hours of inpatient care following a lymph node dissection.[11]

Access to Care

In the current health care environment of concern for cost containment and with the increasing shift toward financial drivers, issues of access to health care resources and due process in determination of access will undoubtedly continue to be important considerations. Lacking societal consensus, there will be a continuing struggle with the notion of justice in allocation of health care resources. Some people will call for a single payer system.

Another continuing dilemma will be whether some level of health care is a right or a privilege. Although there seems to be a minimal level of societal consensus that some level of health care is a right, American society as a whole seems unwilling to endorse further entitlement programs. Although society believes that every person has a right to some health care, there has been reluctance to pay for it. Given the dual mind set on this issue, national political or legislative solutions will probably not be easily fabricated. Lacking the national consensus necessary for major reform legislation, state and local governments will continue to lead the way in health care reform. However, it is likely that national legislation will continue to work on laws to limit the power of managed care entities and to ensure due process in claims.

A New Approach?

Has the four principles approach exhausted its usefulness? If so, what will take its place? Although the answers to these questions are not known, it is known that the four principles approach is least effective in dealing with issues of justice and in critiquing the entire system. The current predominance of issues of justice and the paradigm shift toward a business model suggest that health care is, as Pellegrino[12] has written, in a post-principles crisis. It is not known what the future holds for health care or for medical ethics. For now, the four principles approach is the language of medical ethics. In spite of its limitations, it can help to interpret new ethical directions for physical therapy.

The future of health care may involve more consideration of the fairness of medical determinations and whether due process was provided as notions of what constitutes medical necessity shift. The questions of who is to decide the appropriate level of care and the scope of the factors to be considered in such determinations will pose complex and difficult questions as health care in the twenty-first century is approached.

Triezenberg[13] conducted a study of present and past members of the APTA Judicial Committee to identify their opinions about current and future ethical issues in physical therapy. The panel identified the following 16 current and future ethical issues facing physical therapy:

Current Issues:
1. Overuse of PT services
2. Identification of factors constituting informed consent
3. Protection of a patient's right to confidentiality
4. Justification of appropriate fees charged by PTs
5. Maintaining truth in advertisement
6. PTs maintaining clinical competence
7. Adhering to ethical guidelines for protection of human subjects in PT clinical research

8. Endorsement of products or equipment by PTs who have a financial interest
9. Determining proper training, use, and supervision of support personnel
10. PTs' involvement in business relationships that have potential for exploitation of patients
11. Identification and elimination of fraud in billing
12. Provision of PT services without regard for patients' social or personal characteristics

Future Issues:
13. Responsibility of PTs to respond to environmental issues (pollutants and other health hazards)
14. Duty of PTs to report misconduct of colleagues
15. Need for PTs to define the limits of personal relationships in professional settings
16. Identification of and prevention of sexual and physical abuse of patients in physical therapy (current and future issue)

QUESTIONS AND NOTES FOR FURTHER REFLECTION

1. For discussions of the issues in this chapter, see Rhodes and Miller[14] and Catalano.[15]

2. For a discussion of one APTA chapter's lobbying efforts in support of direct access, see Dahl and Sand.[16]

3. The United States is the only major western country that does not have a single payer system. What are the advantages and disadvantages of a single payer system? Why has the United States resisted this kind of health care system?

4. What are the limitations of the principles approach to ethics? What are the alternatives?

5. What is the current focus of the health care delivery system: cost, quality, or access? In which direction are current forces pushing the system?

6. See Balase et al.[17] for a discussion of some of the implications of telemedicine.

REFERENCES

1. Frederickson HG. The Spirit of Public Administration. San Francisco: Jossey-Bass, 1997;112.
2. Brimer M. The physical therapist as witness. Clin Manage 1987;7:30.

3. Southwick A. The Law of Hospital and Health Care Administration. Ann Arbor, MI: Health Administration Press, 1988;16.
4. Idaho Chapter, APTA sponsor successful legislative health and fitness screening. PT Bull 1997;12:9.
5. Ellis J. Physical therapists storm the Hill to educate legislators about PT profession. PT Bull 1997;12:10.
6. *St. John v. Pope*, 901 S.W.2d 420 (Tex. 1995).
7. Health Insurance Portability and Accountability Act of 1996, Pub. L. 104-91 (H.R. 3103) §192.
8. Physician Insurers Association of America. Telemedicine: An Overview of Applications and Barriers. Rockville, MD: Physician Insurers Association of America, 1996.
9. Telemedicine engenders new malpractice fears. PT Bull 1997;12:18.
10. Newborns' and Mothers' Health Protection Act of 1996. Pub. L. 104-204, §2704, 42 U.S.C. 300gg-4.
11. APTA supports legislation on hospital stays, cancer. PT Bull 1997;12(9):1.
12. Pellegrino ED. The metamorphosis of medical ethics: a 30-year retrospective. JAMA 1993;269:1158–1162.
13. Triezenberg HL. The identification of ethical issues in physical therapy practice. Phys Ther 1996;76:1097–1106.
14. Rhodes A, Miller R. Nursing and the Law (4th ed). Rockville, MD: Aspen, 1984.
15. Catalano J. Ethical and Legal Aspects of Nursing (2nd ed). Springhouse, PA: Springhouse, 1995.
16. Dahl L, Sand M. Effective lobbying at the grass roots level. Clin Manage 1989;9:31
17. Balase E, Jaffrey F, Kuperman G, et al. Electronic communication with patients: evaluation of distance medicine technology. JAMA 1997;278:152.

Glossary

Absolute or actual obligation: As formulated by W.D. Ross, an obligation that cannot be overridden by another obligation. A duty that must always be fulfilled.

Abuse: Affliction of physical pain, injury, or mental anguish, or deprivation of services by a caretaker.

Accountability: The processes by which an individual or group is responsible to another individual or group. Linda and Ezekiel Emanuel delineated three models of accountability: professional, economic, and political.

Americans with Disabilities Act of 1990 (ADA): Requires employers and places of public accommodation to make reasonable modifications to accommodate persons with disabilities.

Administrative law: The regulations and rulings established by administrative agencies and their quasi-judicial hearing bodies in interpreting federal and state statutes.

Advance directive: A legal document that delineates the patient's wishes for future medical care in the event the patient should become decisionally incapacitated. Typically includes living wills and durable powers of attorney. Although advance directives typically refer to documents, they should represent the process of communication and dialogue between family members, loved ones, and care providers.

Any willing provider law: A law that requires managed care organizations to use any provider that meets certain established standards. Any willing provider laws prevent providers from being "locked out" of managed care.

Aristotle (384–322 BC): Greek philosopher who articulated a virtue-based, teleological ethical system.

Ascending order of ethical sensitivity: Edmund Pellegrino's concept that ethical sensitivity increases from its lowest level of simply obeying the law to fulfilling duties and obligations and ultimately to practicing virtue. The ascending order of ethical sensitivity implicitly presumes a virtue-based theory of ethics.

Autonomy: One of the four principles emphasized by Beauchamp and Childress that asserts that people ought to be allowed self-determination. The principle of autonomy describes the right of each person to make decisions regarding his or her behavior and future.

Battery: Legal term designating non-consensual touching.

Beauchamp, Tom L.: Coauthor of *Principles of Biomedical Ethics.* See four principles approach.

Beneficence: One of the four principles emphasized by Beauchamp and Childress that describes the obligation to promote the good or happiness of others. The word *beneficence* comes from the Latin roots *facere* (to do) and *bene* (well).

Boundary: The limits and parameters that define appropriate behavior and interaction between health care provider and patient.

Capitation: Determination of insurance reimbursement in which the health care provider is paid a periodic fee for each service. For example, a physical therapist might be paid $0.30 per life for providing physical therapy services to a particular company for a year.

Casuistry: Ethical position that emphasizes the identification of paradigmatic cases or moral behavior.

Categorical imperative: Theory advanced by Immanuel Kant that individuals ought always to act in such a way that their behavior could become a universal principle. The categorical imperative also states that people should never be treated as means only but rather as ends in themselves.

Chapter ethics committee (CEC): The committee at the chapter level of the American Physical Therapy Association (APTA) that is charged with investigating and recommending action to the Judicial Committee on reported cases of ethical misconduct by members of the APTA.

Childress, James F.: Coauthor of *Principles of Biomedical Ethics.* See four principles approach.

Common law: Legal principles set forth in the decisions of state and federal judges in specific applications.

Common Rule: Rule adopted in 1991 regarding protection of human subjects in all institutions that receive federal funding.

Communitarian ethics: Ethical theory that emphasizes the common good. In medical ethics, this is usually in contrast to an ethical position that emphasizes autonomy.

Comparative justice: That part of the principle of justice that refers to fairness when individuals are compared.

Comparative negligence: Legal theory in which the amount of negligence is apportioned and damages apportioned when both plaintiff and defendant are negligent.

Compensatory justice: Fairness within the context of repayment for past injustice.

Confidentiality: The obligation of health care providers to keep information about patients in confidence and not to reveal such information to persons not authorized to have access to this information.

Consequentialism: The approach to ethics that emphasizes the consequences of actions. Utilitarianism is a form of consequentialism. Utilitarianism attempts to determine the correct course of action by analyzing which action will create the greatest happiness or use. John Stuart Mill and Jeremy Bentham are credited as the founders of utilitarianism.

Context: Context is the situation in which an ethical decision occurs. Context includes familial, cultural, institutional, profession, personal, political, national, and social factors. Richard Zaner has argued that ethical decision making cannot be understood apart from an appreciation of the medical world.

Contributory negligence: The plaintiff is partially responsible for the injury. In some states, if the plaintiff is at all responsible for injury, then he or she may not collect damages. This contrasts to comparative negligence.

Deontology or deontological ethics: The approach to ethics that emphasizes duties and universal rules and laws of human behavior. This approach to ethics is associated with Immanuel Kant.

Descriptive ethics: Field of ethics that uses empirical tools to describe moral behavior. Contrast normative ethics.

Distributive justice: Fairness or equity in the allocation of goods and services.

Do not resuscitate (DNR): A DNR order indicates that medical personnel should not attempt to resuscitate in the event that the patient expires.

Due process: The use of fair processes in adjudicating disputes. Due process is part of the application of the principle of justice.

Durable power of attorney: A legal document that appoints a surrogate decision maker for health care decisions in the event that the patient is incapacitated.

Duties: Moral responsibilities or demands.

Ethic of care: The ethic of care advocates making ethical decisions based on personal relationships rather than on the basis of universal principles of behavior. Carol Gilligan is credited with being the first to propose an ethic of care in *In a Different Voice*, which presented a feminist critique of the moral developmental theory of Lawrence Kohlberg.

Ethics: Field of philosophy that deals with right and wrong human behavior, as well as the basis by which those decisions are made. Rational analysis of morality.

Fee-for-service: Approach to health care reimbursement in which each service rendered has a set fee. Contrast capitation.

Foreseeability: With respect to causation, the extent to which the physical therapist could have projected the outcome of specific behaviors.

Four principles approach: The theory of ethics that emphasizes four intermediate principles: autonomy, beneficence, nonmaleficence, and justice. Tom Beauchamp and James Childress made use of the four principles approach in *Principles of Biomedical Ethics*, published in 1979 and now in its fourth edition.

Four senses of autonomy: Bruce Miller's formulation of autonomy as free action, authenticity, effective deliberation, and moral reflection.

Fraud: Misrepresentation of facts.

Gag rule: A rule established by a health care insurer or provider that prohibits providers from disclosing information, including treatment options, to a patient.

Gatekeeper: Any health care provider who controls access to further health care services or equipment. In managed care, the primary care physician serves as gatekeeper to other services. PTs can serve as gatekeepers to other services. Gatekeeper roles become legally and ethically problematic when they are linked to financial incentives or disincentives to provide or deny care.

Good Samaritan laws: Laws that protect persons who assist victims in an emergency.

Guide for Professional Conduct: APTA document that delineates rules for ethical behavior of the PT. This document also contains applications and interpretations of the *Code of Ethics.*

Guide for Conduct of the Affiliate Member: APTA document that delineates standards of ethical behavior for the physical therapist assistant (PTA). This document also contains rules and interpretations of the *Standards of Ethical Conduct for the Physical Therapist Assistant.*

Health Care Quality Improvement Act (HCQIA): A 1986 federal act that mandates peer review standards and the creation of the National Practitioner Data Bank.

Health Insurance Portability and Accountability Act of 1996 (HIPAA): Federal legislation designed to improve the availability and portability of health care. Among other provisions, HIPAA limits exclusion based on pre-existing conditions and prohibits discrimination based on health status for certain plans.

Immunity: Freedom or protection from prosecution. For example, mandatory reporting abuse laws frequently grant immunity for health care professionals who report suspected abuse.

Informed consent: The process by which providers present information regarding the treatment or research procedure, its risks, benefits, and alternatives and by which patients or subjects agree to participate in treatment or research. Informed consent has at least four elements: disclosure, competence, comprehension, and voluntariness. Although informed consent is frequently viewed as a procedure that culminates in a signed document, informed consent should be viewed as a process in which information is exchanged that forms the foundation for the patient's or subject's decision.

Institutional ethics committee (IEC): A committee within a hospital or health care organization that participates in educating the organization regarding ethical issues, recommending policies and guidelines, and case consultation and review.

Institutional review board (IRB): A committee within an organization that reviews all research proposals for ethical treatment of subjects.

Joint Commission on Accreditation of Healthcare Organizations (JCAHO): A private accrediting agency that establishes standards for hospitals and other health care organizations and determines compliance with those standards. Although compliance with these standards is voluntary, reimbursement and other governmental standards may be driven by compliance with JCAHO.

Judicial Committee (JC): Committee of the APTA appointed by the board of directors that ultimately rules on all ethical complaints brought to the APTA. Decisions of the judicial committee may be appealed to the board of directors.

Justice: One of the four principles emphasized by Beauchamp and Childress that describes the obligation to deal fairly and equally with all persons. This includes the distribution of goods, services, and resources (distributive justice), compensation for injury (compensatory justice), and treating similar cases in a like manner (comparative justice).

Kant, Immanuel (1724–1804): Philosopher who argued that reason provides the basis for universal principles of ethical behavior. Associated with deontological ethics and the categorical imperative.

Kickback: Remuneration for referral for services.

Law: Rules and standards for behavior that are created either by statutes or by common law.

Legal: Behavior that falls within existing laws and regulations.

Liberal individualism: School of ethics emphasizing individual rights that has grown out of John Locke's exposition of the natural rights of human beings.

Living will: A document that specifies those medical interventions that an individual would want or would want withheld should they become incapacitated.

Managed care: Approach to health care delivery that focuses on cost-containment through disincentives to use of health care. These include copayments, point-of-service programs, and using primary care gatekeepers.

Mandatory reporting law: A law that mandates that specified professionals must report suspected cases of abuse. May apply to child abuse, elder abuse, or domestic violence.

Metaethics: Field of ethics concerned with the rational basis for ethical decisions, the nature of good and evil, and the meaning of moral language.

Moral imagination: The use of creativity in resolving ethical problems. This contrasts with deductivism in which principles are rigidly applied to specific situations.

Moral relativism: Position that views differences in ethical judgment as strictly the result of enculturation. Extreme moral relativism denies that there is enduring moral truth. Accordingly, ethical matters cannot be debated and there is no "wrong" ethical position.

Moral developmental approach to ethics: Approach to morality made famous by Lawrence Kohlberg that delineates the six stages of moral development.

Morality: May be used synonymously with ethics. When distinguished from ethics, indicates the entire constellation of customs, moral standards, and rules that guide a particular culture and are internalized by individuals within that culture.

National Practitioner Data Bank: National, computerized data bank for information about adverse actions and medical malpractice created by the Health Care Quality Improvement Act of 1990.

Negligence: Legal principle that includes proving a legal duty, breach of that duty, that the breach caused an injury, and that the injury resulted in damage to the patient.

Noncompete clause: A clause in a contract by which an employee agrees not to accept employment within a specified area following termination of employment for a specified length of time.

Nonmaleficence: One of the four principles emphasized by Beauchamp and Childress that describes the obligation to not harm others. The principle of nonmaleficence is captured by the medical dictum "primum non nocere," which enjoins practitioners to "First, do no harm."

Normative ethics: Field of ethics concerned with what individuals ought to do.

Paternalism: Relationship between patient and provider in which the provider acts as "parent," deciding what is in the patient's best interests without the patient's input or participation. Paternalism compromises the autonomy of the patient.

Patient Self-Determination Act of 1990: Requires that certain entities, including hospitals, nursing homes, hospice programs, and home-health agencies, must inform patients on admission about state laws regarding advance directives.

Pellegrino's four periods of medical ethics: Edmund Pellegrino described medical ethics in four periods: quiescent, principlism, antiprinciplism, and period of crisis.

Prima facie principle: As formulated by W.D. Ross, an obligation or duty that can be overridden by a more important duty. This contrasts with an absolute duty that cannot be overridden by another obligation.

Principle: A guide for moral behavior that is more specific than a theory but more general than a rule. Principles are based on common understandings of morality.

Principlism: See four principles approach.

Procedural document: Document published by the APTA that outlines the actions to be taken when an ethical violation is alleged to have been committed by a member of the APTA.

Profession: A calling that requires specialized knowledge. Traditionally, professions have an organized body of knowledge, a code of ethics, some degree of autonomy, and responsibility to society.

Protection of human subjects: Measures in clinical research with human subjects designed to protect those subjects. Informed consent is one part of protection of human subjects.

Purtilo, Ruth: PT most credited with bringing ethical issues to the attention of the physical therapy profession.

Quinlan case: Landmark case in which the New Jersey Supreme Court ruled that Karen Anne Quinlan's father had the right to act on his daughter's behalf in declining life support. Karen was in a persistive vegetative state.

Rehabilitation Act of 1973: Prohibits denying benefits or discrimination because of handicap or impairment.

Relativism: See moral relativism.

Res ipsa loquitur: Latin for "the thing speaks for itself." With regard to negligence (malpractice), the legal doctrine that says that it is unnecessary to prove causation, as the injury could not have happened without negligence.

Respondeat superior: Legal doctrine in which an employer is responsible for the acts of its employees.

Restraint: Any physical, chemical, or mechanical device that restricts the individual's ability to move freely that the individual cannot remove easily.

Right: Entitlement to act or have others act in a particular way. Legal rights are grounded in the U.S. Constitution, especially the fourteenth amendment with its due process and equal protection clauses.

Ross, W.D. (1877–1971): Philosopher who distinguished prima facie from absolute or actual obligations.

Rule: A guide to moral behavior that is more specific than either an ethical theory or an ethical principle.

Sexual harassment: Unwelcome sexual advances, sexual favors, or other verbal physical conduct of a sexual nature when submission is a requirement of continued employment or when it interferes with work performance or creates a hostile work environment.

Standard of care: In matters of negligence, the standard that bases judgment on whether the therapist acted in a reasonable manner given the circumstances when compared to another prudent therapist.

Statute: A law created by a federal or state legislative act.

Surrogate: One who has legal standing to act on behalf of the patient.

Teleological ethics: Teleological ethics base ethical decisions on "ends." (*Telos* is Greek for "end.") Consequentialism is a teleological ethic because it focuses on the outcomes of actions. Aristotle's virtue-based ethic is also a teleological ethic because it is based on a natural law conception of the appropriate purpose of human activity.

Tort law: Law involving personal injury by another person.

Tort reform: Proposal for change in laws that govern medical malpractice awards.

Utilitarianism: Ethical school that emphasizes the principle of utility or happiness. Utilitarianism advocates seeking the course of action that produces the greatest utility or happiness. Associated with John Stuart Mill (1806–1873) and Jeremy Bentham (1748–1832), utilitarianism is commonly characterized as the greatest good for the greatest number or the greatest balance of good over evil.

Value: Standards of what is desirable or undesirable described as good or bad. Values are learned through the process of socialization.

Virtue or virtue ethics: A personal characteristic, behavior, quality, habit, or disposition that is desirable. Some examples are: fairness, honesty, integrity, compassion, and kindness. Aristotle is famous for his description of the virtues. Different cultures cultivate different virtues. Virtue ethics concentrates on the cultivation of virtues rather than duties or rights. In medical ethics, Pellegrino has argued that virtue-based ethics represents the highest level of ethical sensitivity.

Index